I0704334

Herbal Healing Secrets

Unlock the Power of Herbs to Boost Immunity, Relieve Pain, and Restore Balance Naturally

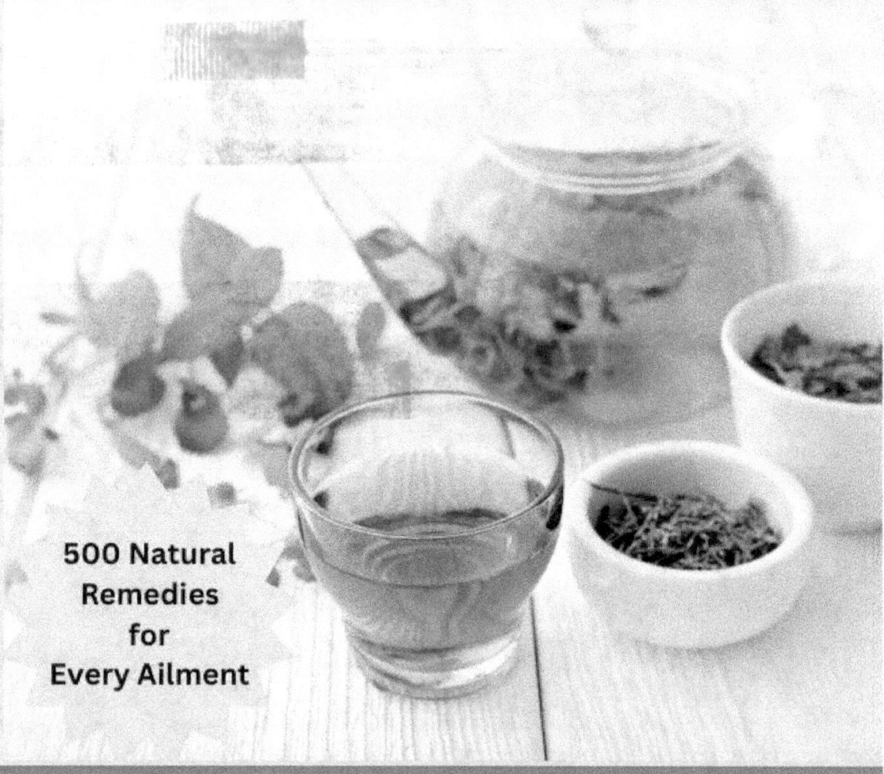

Fiona Smith

Herbal Healing Secrets: 500 Natural Remedies for Every Ailment

"Unlock the Power of Herbs to Boost Immunity, Relieve Pain, and Restore Balance Naturally"

Written By

Fiona Smith

Contents

Introduction

Why Choose Herbal Remedies?

In today's world, where synthetic drugs are often the first response to any health issue, more people are rediscovering the profound healing power of natural remedies. Herbal medicine offers a holistic approach to health, focusing not only on treating symptoms but also on supporting the body's inherent ability to heal.

Herbs have been used across cultures and millennia for their restorative properties. Unlike many modern pharmaceuticals, herbs often come with fewer side effects, are generally more affordable, and are accessible to most people. When you turn to herbs, you're connecting with nature's wisdom, which has been refined and perfected through centuries. Choosing herbal remedies is not just about finding a natural alternative—it's about adopting a lifestyle that values health, balance, and self-care.

The Power of Plants: A Brief History of Herbal Medicine

Herbal medicine has been the foundation of health care in cultures worldwide. From Traditional Chinese Medicine and Ayurveda to Indigenous healing practices, people have relied on plants to heal, nourish, and protect. The oldest recorded herbal traditions date back thousands of years, including Egyptian, Chinese, and Greek medical texts, each detailing the therapeutic properties of plants like garlic, aloe vera, and ginger.

Even today, many pharmaceuticals are derived from plant compounds—aspirin, for instance, was inspired by compounds found in willow bark. In modern times, researchers are continually discovering new plant-based compounds that hold remarkable potential for healing. This legacy of plant-based medicine offers a treasure trove of knowledge, refined over generations, and still relevant in treating the ailments of modern life.

Understanding Holistic Healing: Mind, Body, and Spirit

Holistic healing is rooted in the understanding that our bodies, minds, and spirits are interconnected. Health isn't just the absence of disease; it's a balanced state of well-being that encompasses physical, mental, and emotional aspects. Herbal medicine supports this idea by addressing multiple levels of health simultaneously.

For instance, herbs like lavender can calm the nervous system, which not only eases anxiety but can also improve sleep and digestion—two areas often affected by stress. Adaptogens like ashwagandha can help the body manage stress, supporting mental clarity while also fortifying physical resilience. When you use herbal remedies, you're not just targeting symptoms; you're supporting your body's systems as a whole, helping them to work harmoniously.

This book encourages you to embrace herbal medicine as part of a larger commitment to holistic health. As you explore, you'll discover that herbs can uplift the spirit, strengthen the body, and provide a pathway to a more balanced life.

How to Use This Book for Maximum Benefit

This book is designed to be a user-friendly, comprehensive guide to herbal remedies, structured in a way that's accessible whether you're completely new to herbs or more experienced. Here's a quick roadmap for how to get the most out of it:

1. **Start with the Basics:** The first section introduces foundational concepts, helping you understand how herbs work and the different ways you can prepare and use them. Take time with this part, as it builds the groundwork for deeper knowledge.

2. **Dive into Specific Remedies:** In the middle chapters, you'll find a broad range of remedies for common ailments, organized by health concern. This makes it easy to look up a remedy for something specific, like digestion or sleep, when you need it. Each chapter includes recipes, detailed preparation instructions, and safety information, so you feel confident using each herb.

3. **Experiment and Customize:** Herbal medicine is both an art and a science. As you gain confidence, experiment with different herbs and preparations. The recipes and tips encourage creativity—try new combinations, adjust dosages as you learn how your body responds, and discover your personal favorites.

4. **Explore Advanced Applications and Lifestyle Integration:** The final sections include advanced practices, like creating custom blends and learning about herbs for mental clarity and resilience. You'll also find guidance on incorporating herbs into everyday routines, from using herbs in the kitchen to creating a small herb garden. These tips aim to make herbal medicine a seamless, empowering part of your lifestyle.

Herbal healing is a journey, and this book is your companion along the way. Open yourself to the wisdom of plants, and step into a world of natural healing that has supported humanity for centuries. Whether you're looking to relieve an ailment or simply boost your overall well-being, you'll find inspiration, practical advice, and proven methods in the pages ahead.

Part 1: Foundations of Herbal Medicine

Chapter 1

The Essentials of Herbal Healing

What Is Herbal Medicine?

Herbal medicine is the practice of using plants and plant extracts to support physical, mental, and emotional health. It's a holistic approach that involves harnessing the natural compounds in herbs, flowers, roots, and leaves to restore balance and address health concerns. While modern medicine often focuses on isolated compounds in pharmaceutical drugs, herbal medicine relies on the synergistic effects of multiple compounds within a whole plant, which tend to work in harmony to enhance therapeutic effects and minimize side effects.

Unlike synthetic drugs, which may target a single symptom or bodily system, herbal remedies aim to support the body's natural functions, strengthening its ability to heal itself. For example, chamomile tea can help with relaxation, digestion, and even inflammation. Herbal medicine's versatility, natural basis, and ability to support rather than override the body's natural processes make it an appealing choice for many looking for holistic health options.

How Herbs Work in the Body

Plants contain an incredible variety of active compounds that can influence different systems within the body. These compounds are grouped into several major categories, each with distinct effects:

1. **Alkaloids:** Often found in medicinal plants, alkaloids can be powerful agents. Examples include morphine from poppies and caffeine from coffee beans. In herbs, milder alkaloids provide gentle stimulation or relaxation without drastic side effects.

2. **Flavonoids:** Known for their antioxidant properties, flavonoids help combat free radicals in the body, reducing inflammation and supporting cell health. They're abundant in herbs like chamomile, lemon balm, and hawthorn.

3. **Tannins:** These astringent compounds are helpful for tightening tissues, reducing bleeding, and treating infections. You'll find tannins in herbs like witch hazel, sage, and blackberry leaf.

4. **Terpenes and Terpenoids:** These aromatic compounds give herbs their distinct scents and often have anti-inflammatory, antiviral, or antibacterial effects. Herbs like lavender, rosemary, and peppermint are rich in terpenes.

5. **Glycosides and Saponins:** These compounds help stimulate different organs or processes, such as digestion, metabolism, or detoxification. Licorice and ginseng contain beneficial saponins that help boost immune function and regulate stress response.

When you use herbal remedies, these active compounds interact with the body's biochemistry to support healing, alleviate discomfort, or balance bodily functions. Unlike isolated chemical compounds, herbal medicine typically uses the whole plant, allowing for multiple therapeutic effects and a more balanced interaction with the body.

The Science Behind Plant-Based Healing

In recent years, the science supporting plant-based healing has grown significantly, validating what many traditional practitioners have known for centuries. Modern studies reveal that the healing properties of plants go beyond folklore and are based on biochemistry. Here's a look at some scientific principles behind herbal medicine:

1. **Synergy of Compounds:** Research shows that the therapeutic power of plants often comes from the synergy of multiple compounds. For example, while curcumin is the main active compound in turmeric, studies suggest it's more effective when combined with other curcuminoids naturally present in the plant. This synergy enhances bioavailability and effectiveness.

2. **Bioavailability and Body-Friendly Action:** Many plant compounds are naturally bioavailable, meaning they're easy for the body to absorb and use. Additionally, the structure of plant compounds often closely resembles human body biochemistry, which allows for gentle, body-friendly healing without overwhelming the system.

3. **Adaptogens and Body Balance:** Certain herbs, known as adaptogens, are scientifically recognized for their ability to help the body adapt to stress. Ashwagandha, rhodiola, and holy basil are examples of adaptogens that help regulate stress hormones, support mental clarity, and improve energy without stimulating side effects.

4. **Clinical Research and Efficacy:** Herbs like ginger, garlic, and ginkgo biloba have been extensively studied in clinical trials, validating their use for ailments like nausea, heart health, and cognitive support. As researchers continue to investigate plant-based compounds, more scientific evidence emerges to support the benefits of herbs in managing chronic conditions and promoting general wellness.

5. **Preventative Health:** Unlike many pharmaceuticals, herbal medicine emphasizes preventative care. Many herbs support the body's immune defenses, help detoxify, and nourish vital organs, creating a foundation of health that can help prevent illness. Studies have shown that regularly consuming antioxidant-rich herbs like

rosemary, turmeric, and green tea can protect cells, reduce inflammation, and lower
the risk of chronic disease.

By understanding how herbs interact with the body and how their natural compounds can
support our health, we gain deeper respect for plant-based healing. Throughout this book,
you'll learn about specific herbs, their uses, and evidence-based insights that bridge
traditional wisdom with modern science. Each chapter builds on this foundation, guiding
you to incorporate herbal medicine into your daily life and achieve a new level of health and
well-being.

Embrace this journey, and discover how herbal healing can transform your approach to
health, offering solutions rooted in nature and proven by science.

Chapter 2

Getting Started: Building Your Herbal Healing Kit

Essential Herbs for Every Home

Creating a well-rounded herbal healing kit starts with selecting versatile, effective herbs that address a wide range of common health concerns. Here's a list of essential herbs that are beginner-friendly, widely available, and highly effective:

1. **Chamomile** – Known for its calming properties, chamomile helps with relaxation, sleep, and digestive discomfort. It's safe for all ages and can be used as a tea, compress, or skin rinse.

2. **Peppermint** – A go-to herb for digestive health, headaches, and respiratory relief. Peppermint can be used in tea, as an essential oil, or in topical applications to soothe muscles and clear the sinuses.

3. **Ginger** – Known for its anti-inflammatory and warming properties, ginger helps with nausea, muscle pain, and circulatory health. Fresh ginger root is versatile and can be used in teas, tinctures, or as a topical poultice.

4. **Lavender** – A powerful herb for relaxation and skin health, lavender is beneficial in teas, aromatherapy, and topical treatments. It also has antiseptic properties and can be used in DIY skin remedies.

5. **Echinacea** – A natural immune booster, echinacea is essential for colds, flu, and infection prevention. It's commonly used in teas, capsules, or tinctures during cold and flu season.

6. **Turmeric** – Known for its potent anti-inflammatory effects, turmeric supports joint health, digestion, and liver detoxification. It can be used in food, capsules, or as a tincture for regular wellness support.

7. **Calendula** – Ideal for skin healing, calendula is gentle yet effective for wounds, rashes, and minor cuts. It can be made into creams, oils, or tinctures and has antibacterial and anti-inflammatory properties.

Each of these herbs offers a range of health benefits, making them versatile additions to any home herbal kit. As you gain confidence, you can expand your collection to include herbs specific to your personal health needs.

Tools, Tinctures, and Preparations

To prepare and use herbal remedies, a few simple tools will make your work more efficient and your remedies more effective:

1. **Basic Tools:**

   - **Mortar and Pestle**: For grinding fresh herbs into pastes or powders.

   - **Herb Grinder**: Useful for dried herbs that need to be ground before use.

   - **Strainers or Cheesecloth**: For filtering out plant material when making teas, tinctures, or infusions.

   - **Amber Glass Jars or Bottles**: Essential for storing tinctures, oils, and salves; amber glass protects herbs from light and keeps them potent longer.

   - **Mason Jars**: Handy for steeping teas, making tinctures, or infusions.

   - **Measuring Spoons and Dropper Bottles**: For accurate dosing of tinctures and essential oils.

2. **Types of Herbal Preparations:**

   - **Teas and Infusions**: Simple to prepare and highly effective, teas and infusions involve steeping herbs in hot water to extract their beneficial compounds. Infusions are ideal for soft herbs (like leaves and flowers), while decoctions work better for tougher materials like roots and bark.

- o **Tinctures**: Alcohol-based extracts that concentrate the active compounds in herbs, making them potent and long-lasting. Tinctures are convenient, with a few drops providing a concentrated dose.

- o **Oils and Salves**: Herb-infused oils are used for topical applications, while salves add beeswax to make a spreadable balm. Both are great for skin issues, sore muscles, and minor wounds.

- o **Poultices and Compresses**: For more immediate relief, crushed or ground herbs are applied directly to the skin and covered with a cloth. Poultices are effective for bruises, swelling, and inflammation.

Understanding these preparation methods will allow you to create custom remedies suited to your unique health needs and preferences.

How to Source, Grow, and Store Herbs Safely

Quality is essential in herbal medicine, as herbs need to retain their potency for maximum effectiveness. Here's a guide on sourcing, growing, and storing herbs for your herbal kit:

1. **Sourcing Herbs:**

   - o **Reputable Suppliers**: Choose certified organic suppliers that offer sustainably sourced herbs. Look for labels like "organic" or "wildcrafted" to ensure you're getting high-quality products.

   - o **Farmers Markets and Health Stores**: Local markets and health food stores often carry fresh, organic herbs. This is a good option for herbs that you want to buy fresh.

   - o **Online Herbal Retailers**: There are reputable online herbal stores specializing in high-quality, sustainably harvested herbs. Ensure they have transparent sourcing and quality standards.

2. **Growing Your Own Herbs:**

   - o **Start with Hardy, Low-Maintenance Herbs**: Herbs like mint, rosemary, thyme, and basil are easy to grow and work well in containers. They thrive indoors and out, making them great starter plants.

- o **Create a Dedicated Herb Garden**: For those with outdoor space, an herb garden can be a rewarding way to ensure you have fresh, organic herbs year-round. Select herbs suited to your climate, and consider rotating them to ensure soil health.

- o **Harvest Carefully**: When harvesting, only take what you need, leaving enough plant material for regrowth. Morning harvests retain the most essential oils, especially in flowering herbs like lavender or chamomile.

3. **Storing Herbs for Longevity and Potency:**

- o **Drying Herbs**: To store herbs long-term, drying is essential. Hang small bundles of herbs upside down in a dark, dry space with good airflow. Once fully dry, crumble them into jars.

- o **Use Airtight Containers**: Dried herbs should be stored in airtight containers, ideally in dark glass jars to prevent exposure to light and moisture.

- o **Label and Date Your Herbs**: To keep track of potency, label each container with the herb name and date of storage. Most dried herbs remain effective for 6-12 months if stored properly.

- o **Keep Away from Heat and Light**: Store herbs in a cool, dark place to preserve their healing properties. Avoiding exposure to direct sunlight and high humidity will help prevent the herbs from losing potency.

By building a well-stocked herbal healing kit and learning the essentials of herbal preparations, you're laying the groundwork for a successful journey into natural medicine. As you continue exploring, remember that creating and using herbal remedies is an evolving process. Enjoy the satisfaction of crafting your own remedies, discovering the healing power of plants, and developing your personalized approach to holistic wellness.

Chapter 3

Herbal Preparation Basics

Types of Herbal Preparations (Teas, Tinctures, Salves, etc.)

Different types of herbal preparations allow you to harness the healing benefits of herbs in a way that suits both your lifestyle and specific health needs. Each preparation method has its own advantages, making certain herbs more effective depending on how they're used. Here's an overview of the most common types of herbal preparations:

1. **Teas and Infusions**

   - **Infusions** involve steeping soft herbs, such as leaves and flowers, in hot water for about 10-15 minutes to extract their therapeutic compounds. Common infusion herbs include chamomile, lemon balm, and peppermint.

   - **Decoctions** are used for tougher parts of the plant, like roots, bark, and seeds, which need a longer simmering time (20-40 minutes) to release their medicinal properties. Examples include ginger root, burdock root, and cinnamon bark.

   - **How to Use**: Teas are easy to incorporate into daily routines and are especially effective for mild issues, like digestion, relaxation, and hydration.

2. **Tinctures**

   - **What They Are**: Tinctures are concentrated liquid extracts made by soaking herbs in alcohol (or sometimes glycerin or vinegar for a non-alcoholic version) for several weeks. This process draws out the active compounds in herbs and preserves them for long-term use.

- o **Benefits**: Tinctures are potent, quick-acting, and require only a small dosage—often just a few drops. They're particularly useful for immune support, stress relief, and other needs that benefit from consistent dosing.

- o **How to Use**: Tinctures are taken orally, either directly under the tongue for rapid absorption or diluted in water.

3. **Herbal Oils and Salves**

- o **Herbal Oils**: Infused oils are made by steeping herbs in a carrier oil (like olive or coconut oil) to absorb their therapeutic properties. These oils are commonly used for massage, skin treatments, and as the base for making salves.

- o **Salves**: Adding beeswax to herbal oils creates a thicker balm, which can be applied to the skin to soothe rashes, wounds, and inflammation. Calendula, lavender, and arnica are popular herbs for salves.

- o **How to Use**: Oils and salves are applied topically, making them ideal for muscle aches, skin healing, and insect bites.

4. **Poultices and Compresses**

- o **Poultices**: These are soft herbal pastes made by crushing fresh or dried herbs and applying them directly to the skin. They're especially effective for swelling, bruises, and localized pain.

- o **Compresses**: Made by soaking a cloth in a strong herbal infusion or decoction, compresses are placed on the skin to relieve inflammation, soothe aches, and help with skin conditions.

- o **How to Use**: Both methods are applied to the skin and are effective for localized, external issues, such as sprains, wounds, or sore muscles.

5. **Capsules and Powders**

- o For herbs with a strong taste or for people who prefer not to use alcohol-based tinctures, powdered herbs can be encapsulated for easy, measured dosing. Common examples include turmeric, garlic, and ashwagandha.

- o **How to Use**: Capsules are swallowed with water, making them convenient for daily supplementation.

Dosage Guidelines and Safety Precautions

When using herbal remedies, understanding proper dosage and safety guidelines is essential. Unlike pharmaceutical drugs, which are standardized, herbs vary in potency and effects depending on the species, growing conditions, and preparation methods. Here are some general guidelines for safe herbal usage:

1. **Dosage Guidelines**

   - o **Teas and Infusions**: Generally, 1-2 cups per day is safe for most herbs, with some stronger herbs limited to 1 cup.

   - o **Tinctures**: The standard dose for tinctures is around 15-30 drops, taken 2-3 times a day, depending on the herb's potency. Always start with the lowest effective dose and adjust based on personal response.

   - o **Capsules**: Follow the manufacturer's dosage recommendations, typically 1-2 capsules per day, depending on the herb and the reason for use.

   - o **Topicals**: For oils, salves, and poultices, there's no strict dosage, but always test a small amount on the skin first to check for reactions.

2. **Safety Precautions**

   - o **Start Slowly**: Introduce one herb at a time, especially if you're new to herbal remedies. This allows you to monitor for any side effects or allergic reactions.

   - o **Know the Herb's Effects**: Some herbs, such as valerian, can cause drowsiness, while others like ginseng can be stimulating. Understanding each herb's specific actions helps you avoid unintended effects.

   - o **Pregnancy, Nursing, and Children**: Consult a healthcare provider before using herbs during pregnancy, nursing, or for young children. Some herbs, like peppermint or sage, may be safe for adults but not for small children or during pregnancy.

- **Interactions with Medications**: If you're taking prescription medications, talk to your doctor before introducing herbal remedies, as some herbs can interact with pharmaceuticals (e.g., St. John's Wort with antidepressants).

Step-by-Step Guide to Making Herbal Remedies at Home

Let's walk through the steps to make some common herbal remedies at home, using simple ingredients and techniques.

1. **Making Herbal Tea (Infusion)**

   - **Ingredients**: 1-2 tsp of dried herbs (or 1-2 tbsp of fresh herbs), 1 cup boiling water.

   - **Instructions**: Place herbs in a mug or teapot, pour over boiling water, cover, and let steep for 10-15 minutes. Strain before drinking.

   - **Storage**: Herbal teas are best enjoyed fresh. If you need to store, refrigerate and consume within 24 hours.

2. **Preparing a Tincture**

   - **Ingredients**: Dried herbs, 80-100 proof vodka or brandy, glass jar with a lid.

   - **Instructions**: Fill a glass jar 1/3 full with dried herbs, then pour vodka until the jar is nearly full. Seal tightly and store in a dark place for 4-6 weeks, shaking daily. Afterward, strain out the herbs and store the tincture in a dropper bottle.

   - **Storage**: Tinctures can last for years when stored in a cool, dark place.

3. **Making a Salve**

   - **Ingredients**: 1 cup herb-infused oil (like calendula or lavender), 1 oz beeswax.

- o **Instructions**: Heat the oil in a double boiler, then add beeswax until melted. Pour into jars or tins and allow it to cool and harden.

  - o **Storage**: Store salves in a cool place, where they'll last up to a year.

4. **Creating a Poultice**

   - o **Ingredients**: Fresh or dried herbs, hot water, gauze or clean cloth.

   - o **Instructions**: Crush fresh herbs or rehydrate dried herbs with hot water. Place the herbs directly on the skin or wrap them in gauze, applying to the affected area for 15-20 minutes.

   - o **Storage**: Poultices are made for immediate use and should not be stored.

With these foundational recipes and guidelines, you'll be able to confidently prepare a range of herbal remedies that are safe, effective, and personalized to your needs. As you gain experience, you'll find the process becomes second nature, empowering you to take charge of your health in a natural and sustainable way.

Part 2: Ailment-Specific Herbal Remedies

Chapter 4

Immune System Boosters

A strong immune system is the foundation of good health, defending us against colds, flu, and infections. Herbs can play a significant role in both preventing illness and speeding up recovery when sickness strikes. In this chapter, we'll explore powerful immune-boosting herbs, how they work, and how to use them effectively.

Fighting Colds, Flu, and Infections Naturally

When a cold or flu hits, herbal remedies can offer relief from symptoms and help the body recover faster. Here are some effective herbs for immune support during sickness:

1. **Elderberry** – Known for its antiviral properties, elderberry is highly effective in reducing the duration and severity of colds and flu. Elderberry works by blocking viruses from attaching to cells, making it harder for infections to spread.

2. **Echinacea** – A powerful immune stimulant, echinacea is best taken at the first sign of illness. It helps increase white blood cell production, strengthening the body's response to infection. Studies have shown echinacea can reduce cold duration when taken early.

3. **Garlic** – A potent antimicrobial, garlic is effective against bacteria, viruses, and fungi. Rich in allicin, garlic is particularly useful for respiratory infections and general immune support. Eating it raw or in capsules maximizes its benefits.

4. **Ginger** – This warming herb supports the immune system and has strong anti-inflammatory properties. Ginger is also effective for soothing sore throats and helping with congestion.

5. **Licorice Root** – Licorice root helps relieve sore throats, reduce inflammation, and act as an expectorant for respiratory conditions. Its antiviral properties make it an excellent addition to cold and flu remedies.

Herbs for Prevention and Fast Recovery

In addition to fighting infections, certain herbs help strengthen the immune system for long-term resilience. Regularly incorporating these herbs into your routine can make your body more resistant to illness:

1. **Astragalus** – This adaptogenic herb is known for its immune-strengthening and anti-inflammatory effects. Astragalus boosts immune function over time, making it ideal for prevention. It's often used in soups, teas, or as a tincture.

2. **Reishi Mushroom** – Reishi is a medicinal mushroom with immune-modulating properties. It enhances immune response while reducing inflammation, making it helpful for people prone to frequent colds. Reishi can be consumed as a tea, tincture, or in capsule form.

3. **Turmeric** – The active compound in turmeric, curcumin, has powerful anti-inflammatory and antioxidant effects. Regular use of turmeric can help reduce susceptibility to infections and keep inflammation in check.

4. **Rosehip** – Packed with vitamin C, rosehip is excellent for immune support. It's particularly helpful during cold and flu season when the body's vitamin C needs are higher. Rosehip can be used in teas, syrups, or added to smoothies.

5. **Lemon Balm** – Known for its antiviral effects, lemon balm supports the immune system and helps prevent infections. It's also calming, making it a great addition to teas for relaxation and wellness.

Recipe: Elderberry Syrup for Immune Health

Elderberry syrup is a delicious, potent immune booster that's safe for adults and children. It's particularly useful during cold and flu season, as elderberries are packed with antioxidants and compounds that inhibit viral replication. Here's a simple recipe to make your own elderberry syrup at home.

Ingredients:

- 1 cup dried elderberries (or 2 cups fresh elderberries)
- 4 cups water
- 1-2 cinnamon sticks
- 1 tbsp fresh ginger root, grated
- 5-6 whole cloves
- 1 cup raw honey

Instructions:

1. **Simmer the Herbs**: In a saucepan, combine the elderberries, water, cinnamon, ginger, and cloves. Bring to a boil, then reduce heat and let it simmer for 45 minutes, or until the liquid is reduced by half.
2. **Strain and Cool**: Remove the pan from heat and let it cool slightly. Strain the mixture through a fine mesh strainer or cheesecloth into a clean bowl, pressing the berries to extract all the juice.
3. **Add Honey**: Once the liquid has cooled to lukewarm (so it doesn't destroy the honey's beneficial enzymes), stir in the honey until fully dissolved. Adjust the amount of honey based on taste preferences.
4. **Bottle and Store**: Pour the syrup into a glass bottle or jar, and store it in the refrigerator. It will last for up to 2 months when refrigerated.

Dosage:

- For adults: 1 tablespoon daily for prevention, or 1 tablespoon every 2-3 hours during an active cold or flu.
- For children (age 1 and up): 1 teaspoon daily for prevention, or 1 teaspoon every 2-3 hours when sick.

Incorporating these herbs and remedies into your lifestyle will not only help you recover faster from colds and infections but will also build your immune system's resilience. From quick-acting remedies like elderberry syrup to preventive herbs like astragalus and reishi, herbal medicine offers safe, effective tools to support your body's natural defenses. By regularly using immune-boosting herbs and nourishing your body with natural compounds, you're actively enhancing your body's capacity to stay healthy, season after season.

Chapter 5

Digestive Health

The digestive system is at the core of overall health, affecting energy, immunity, and even mood. Many herbs offer safe, effective relief from digestive discomforts like bloating, nausea, and indigestion. They can also support gut health, promote balance in the microbiome, and repair the digestive lining. This chapter explores herbal remedies for common digestive issues, approaches to healing the gut, and a simple recipe for a soothing Peppermint and Ginger Tonic.

Remedies for Bloating, Nausea, and Indigestion

Digestive discomfort is common, but herbs can provide gentle and immediate relief without the side effects of conventional medications. Here are some of the most effective herbs for addressing specific digestive issues:

1. **Peppermint** – A go-to for relieving gas and bloating, peppermint relaxes the muscles of the gastrointestinal tract, making it particularly effective for bloating, cramps, and irritable bowel syndrome (IBS). It can be consumed as a tea or used as an essential oil in diluted form.

2. **Ginger** – Known for its anti-nausea and anti-inflammatory effects, ginger is ideal for upset stomachs, indigestion, and morning sickness. It stimulates digestion and promotes bile production, helping to alleviate indigestion and gas.

3. **Fennel** – A natural carminative, fennel is excellent for reducing gas, bloating, and cramping. It helps relax the intestinal muscles and promotes the expulsion of gas, making it effective after meals. Fennel seeds can be chewed or steeped in hot water for tea.

4. **Chamomile** – Chamomile has calming properties that ease tension in the digestive tract, making it effective for stress-related indigestion and gas. Its anti-inflammatory properties also soothe the stomach lining.

5. **Slippery Elm** – This mucilaginous herb coats the digestive tract, providing relief from irritation, heartburn, and acid reflux. Slippery elm is especially beneficial for conditions like gastritis and ulcerative colitis, where gut lining protection is needed.

6. **Licorice Root (DGL)** – Deglycyrrhizinated licorice (DGL) is a soothing, anti-inflammatory herb that helps reduce stomach acid and repair the mucosal lining, making it effective for ulcers and acid reflux. It's typically taken in tablet or chewable form before meals.

Healing the Gut with Herbal Medicine

Chronic digestive issues often stem from an imbalance in gut health. Restoring balance and repairing the gut lining is essential for long-term relief and wellness. The following herbs can aid in gut healing and promote a healthy microbiome:

1. **Marshmallow Root** – High in mucilage, marshmallow root coats the digestive tract and provides soothing relief for inflammation and irritation. It helps protect the gut lining, supporting healing from conditions like leaky gut syndrome and gastritis.

2. **Calendula** – Known for its anti-inflammatory and antimicrobial properties, calendula helps heal the gut lining and reduce inflammation. It's particularly helpful for ulcerative colitis, Crohn's disease, and IBS.

3. **Aloe Vera** – Aloe vera juice has soothing properties and helps reduce inflammation in the gut, providing relief for people with acid reflux, IBS, and inflammatory bowel diseases. It promotes healing of the gut lining and is gentle on the digestive system.

4. **Turmeric** – The active compound in turmeric, curcumin, has potent anti-inflammatory and antioxidant effects that support overall gut health and reduce inflammation in the digestive tract. It's beneficial for conditions like colitis, leaky gut, and IBS.

5. **Oregano Oil** – Known for its antimicrobial properties, oregano oil can help address bacterial overgrowth in the gut, such as SIBO (small intestine bacterial overgrowth). It's effective against harmful bacteria, fungi, and parasites without disrupting the gut's beneficial microbes.

6. **L-Glutamine** – Though technically an amino acid, L-glutamine is a key component for gut healing. It helps repair and rebuild the mucosal lining of the intestines, making it ideal for those with leaky gut syndrome or chronic digestive inflammation.

Recipe: Peppermint and Ginger Tonic

This soothing tonic combines the digestive benefits of peppermint and ginger to relieve bloating, gas, and nausea. It's a refreshing, effective remedy that can be enjoyed hot or cold.

Ingredients:

- 1 tsp dried peppermint leaves (or 1 tbsp fresh peppermint leaves)

- 1 tsp grated fresh ginger root (or ½ tsp dried ginger powder)

- 1 cup boiling water

- 1 tsp honey or lemon (optional, for flavor)

Instructions:

1. **Steep the Herbs**: Place the peppermint and ginger in a teapot or heatproof mug. Pour the boiling water over the herbs, cover, and let steep for 10-15 minutes.

2. **Strain and Sweeten**: Strain out the herbs, add honey or lemon if desired, and enjoy warm. For a cooling tonic, let it cool and serve over ice.

3. **Optional**: To make a larger batch, double or triple the ingredients, store in the refrigerator, and drink as needed. This tonic can last for up to 3 days when refrigerated.

Usage:

- Drink 1 cup after meals to ease digestion, or sip slowly at the onset of bloating, nausea, or indigestion.

By using herbal remedies for common digestive complaints, you can achieve natural, lasting relief from symptoms while supporting overall gut health. Whether you're looking to soothe occasional indigestion or heal chronic digestive issues, herbs like peppermint, ginger, and marshmallow root can be powerful allies. In addition to alleviating symptoms, these remedies help restore balance, allowing you to maintain digestive health and overall wellness.

Chapter 6

Stress and Anxiety Relief

Life's pressures can lead to stress, anxiety, and even sleep difficulties. Fortunately, many herbs are known for their calming effects on the mind and body, offering relief without the side effects of synthetic medications. In this chapter, we'll cover some of the best herbs for calming anxiety and stress, enhancing sleep quality, and promoting relaxation. Plus, you'll find a simple recipe for Chamomile and Lavender Sleep Tea to help you unwind at the end of the day.

Calming Herbs for Anxiety, Stress, and Overwhelm

These calming herbs provide gentle yet effective relief from stress and anxiety, helping you feel balanced and grounded. Whether you're looking for something to manage daily stress or occasional overwhelming feelings, these herbs can be a great addition to your wellness routine:

1. **Ashwagandha** – This adaptogenic herb is renowned for reducing stress by balancing cortisol levels and supporting adrenal health. Ashwagandha helps the body adapt to stress, promoting a calm, steady energy rather than sedation, making it ideal for daytime use.

2. **Passionflower** – Passionflower has long been used as a natural remedy for anxiety, as it increases gamma-aminobutyric acid (GABA) in the brain, helping to calm the nervous system. Passionflower is helpful for both stress and insomnia, making it useful when taken in the evening.

3. **Lemon Balm** – Lemon balm is a calming herb that reduces stress, eases anxiety, and lifts mood. Its mild sedative properties make it ideal for calming the mind and relaxing the body. It can be enjoyed as a tea or taken as a tincture.

4. **Valerian Root** – Known for its sedative effects, valerian root is a strong herb for anxiety, stress, and sleep troubles. It helps calm the nervous system and reduce restlessness but should be used primarily at night, as it may cause drowsiness.

5. **Holy Basil (Tulsi)** – Another adaptogen, holy basil helps the body cope with stress and reduces anxiety. It supports emotional balance and can enhance clarity and focus, making it useful for daytime stress relief.

6. **Skullcap** – Skullcap is a gentle nervous system tonic that reduces muscle tension and promotes relaxation. It's particularly helpful for people who feel stress physically, such as in tense shoulders or clenched jaws.

Natural Sleep Aids and Relaxation Tips

A good night's sleep is essential for managing stress and maintaining a balanced mood. Here are some herbal sleep aids and tips for creating a relaxing bedtime routine that promotes restful, restorative sleep:

1. **Chamomile** – Chamomile is one of the most well-known herbs for relaxation and sleep. Its mild sedative effects help ease anxiety and promote calm, making it a perfect herb for a pre-sleep tea or bath.

2. **Lavender** – Lavender is well-documented for its soothing effects on the nervous system. Inhaling lavender essential oil or drinking it as a tea can reduce anxiety, promote relaxation, and help with insomnia.

3. **California Poppy** – California poppy is a gentle, non-habit-forming sleep aid that promotes calm and helps with sleep onset. It's particularly helpful for those who have trouble falling asleep due to an active mind.

4. **Magnesium-Rich Herbs** – Magnesium helps regulate sleep patterns and relax muscles, promoting restful sleep. Herbs high in magnesium, like oat straw and nettle, can help with relaxation and support overall nervous system health.

5. **Relaxation Tips for Better Sleep**:

    o   **Create a Routine**: Going to bed and waking up at the same time each day can improve sleep quality. A consistent routine helps regulate your body's internal clock.

    o   **Limit Stimulants**: Avoid caffeine and electronic screens at least an hour before bed. Stimulants can disrupt the body's natural ability to relax and wind down.

    o   **Create a Relaxing Environment**: Dim the lights, play soothing music, or diffuse calming essential oils like lavender or cedarwood to prepare your mind and body for rest.

Recipe: Chamomile and Lavender Sleep Tea

This gentle tea combines chamomile and lavender to help ease stress, calm the mind, and promote deep sleep. It's naturally caffeine-free, making it a perfect choice to drink before bed.

Ingredients:

- 1 tsp dried chamomile flowers
- ½ tsp dried lavender buds
- 1 tsp dried lemon balm leaves (optional, for added calm)
- 1 cup boiling water
- Honey (optional, to taste)

Instructions:

1. **Combine the Herbs**: Place chamomile, lavender, and lemon balm (if using) in a teapot or mug.

2. **Steep the Tea**: Pour the boiling water over the herbs, cover, and let steep for 10 minutes.

3. **Strain and Serve**: Strain the tea into a cup, add honey if desired, and enjoy warm.

Usage:

- Drink 1 cup of this tea about 30 minutes before bedtime to help relax the body and mind.

Incorporating calming herbs and relaxation practices into your routine can have a profound effect on reducing stress, easing anxiety, and improving sleep quality. With the gentle power of herbs like chamomile, lavender, and ashwagandha, you can restore balance, manage stress, and cultivate a sense of calm and well-being. Over time, these natural remedies will help your body and mind develop resilience, allowing you to navigate life's challenges with greater ease and peace.

Chapter 7

Pain Management and Inflammation Reduction

Pain and inflammation, whether acute or chronic, can significantly affect our quality of life. Conventional pain medications often come with side effects, but herbal remedies can provide effective, natural relief without unwanted risks. In this chapter, we'll cover some of the most powerful herbal painkillers, anti-inflammatory herbs for managing chronic pain, and a versatile recipe for a Turmeric and Ginger Anti-Inflammatory Paste.

Herbal Painkillers for Headaches, Muscle Pain, and Joint Relief

Herbs offer gentle but effective options for pain relief, addressing everything from headaches and sore muscles to joint pain. Here are some of the best herbs to consider for natural pain management:

1. **Willow Bark** – Often called "nature's aspirin," willow bark contains salicin, a compound that the body converts into salicylic acid. It's effective for relieving headaches, back pain, and arthritis. Willow bark can be taken as a tea, tincture, or capsule.

2. **Devil's Claw** – Native to southern Africa, devil's claw has strong analgesic and anti-inflammatory effects, making it effective for joint pain, arthritis, and lower back pain. It can be taken as a supplement or in a tea form.

3. **Cayenne (Capsaicin)** – The active compound in cayenne, capsaicin, works by reducing the intensity of pain signals in the body. When applied topically, cayenne can relieve muscle pain, joint pain, and neuropathic pain, often associated with conditions like fibromyalgia.

4. **White Willow** – Similar to willow bark, white willow is another natural source of salicin and is helpful for reducing headaches and muscle soreness. It's especially beneficial for those with tension headaches and mild joint pain.

5. **Arnica** – While not typically ingested, arnica is widely used in topical preparations for pain relief. It's effective for bruises, sprains, and muscle pain when applied as a gel, cream, or oil. Arnica works by reducing inflammation and promoting blood circulation to the affected area.

6. **Clove** – Known for its strong analgesic properties, clove is particularly useful for dental pain. Clove oil can be applied directly to a sore tooth or diluted and applied to other areas of pain for temporary relief.

Anti-Inflammatory Herbs for Chronic Pain

Chronic pain is often tied to inflammation in the body. These anti-inflammatory herbs can reduce pain over time by targeting inflammation at the source, making them ideal for conditions like arthritis, fibromyalgia, and general inflammatory disorders:

1. **Turmeric** – Turmeric is one of the most potent anti-inflammatory herbs available, thanks to curcumin, its active compound. Regular use of turmeric can help reduce chronic pain associated with arthritis and other inflammatory conditions. Turmeric is most effective when combined with black pepper, which enhances curcumin absorption.

2. **Ginger** – Ginger's anti-inflammatory properties are well-suited for managing pain from conditions like osteoarthritis, rheumatoid arthritis, and muscle soreness. It can be consumed as a tea, added to meals, or taken in supplement form for consistent relief.

3. **Boswellia (Frankincense)** – Boswellia is highly effective for reducing inflammation in conditions like arthritis and inflammatory bowel disease. Its anti-inflammatory properties target specific inflammatory pathways, helping with chronic pain and stiffness.

4. **Rosemary** – Known for its antioxidant and anti-inflammatory effects, rosemary is particularly useful for muscle pain and stiffness. It can be consumed as a tea or applied topically to sore muscles and joints.

5. **Green Tea** – Rich in antioxidants called catechins, green tea reduces inflammation and oxidative stress in the body. Drinking green tea regularly can help alleviate chronic pain, especially when associated with inflammatory conditions.

6. **St. John's Wort** – Often used for nerve pain, St. John's Wort has anti-inflammatory properties that can alleviate conditions like sciatica, shingles, and fibromyalgia. It's most effective when taken as an oil or tincture.

Recipe: Turmeric and Ginger Anti-Inflammatory Paste

This versatile paste combines turmeric and ginger's powerful anti-inflammatory properties, making it an excellent addition to your daily routine. You can use it in smoothies, teas, or even as a base for golden milk to help reduce chronic inflammation and manage pain.

Ingredients:

- ½ cup turmeric powder

- 2 tbsp grated fresh ginger (or 1 tbsp dried ginger powder)

- 1-2 tsp black pepper (to enhance turmeric absorption)

- ½ cup water

- 1 tbsp coconut oil (optional, for a creamier texture)

Instructions:

1. **Combine and Heat**: In a small saucepan, mix the turmeric powder, ginger, black pepper, and water. Stir well to combine.

2. **Simmer**: Place the saucepan over low heat and let the mixture simmer, stirring frequently, until it thickens to a paste consistency. This should take about 7-10 minutes.

3. **Add Coconut Oil**: Once the paste has thickened, remove it from the heat and add coconut oil if desired. Stir until fully combined.

4. **Store**: Transfer the paste to a glass jar and store it in the refrigerator for up to two weeks.

Usage:

- **Golden Milk**: Stir a teaspoon of the paste into warm milk (dairy or plant-based), add honey if desired, and enjoy as a soothing evening drink.

- **Smoothies**: Add a teaspoon of the paste to your morning smoothie for an anti-inflammatory boost.

- **Teas and Soups**: Mix a small amount into tea or soups for added flavor and anti-inflammatory benefits.

By incorporating these herbal remedies into your routine, you can find relief from both acute and chronic pain without the risks of synthetic medications. From the immediate pain-relieving effects of herbs like willow bark and arnica to the long-term benefits of anti-inflammatory herbs like turmeric and ginger, nature offers effective, accessible solutions. By addressing the root causes of inflammation and pain, these remedies support your body's healing process and enhance your quality of life naturally and sustainably.

Chapter 8

Skin Health and Natural Beauty

The skin is our largest organ and serves as a protective barrier, reflecting our overall health and well-being. Many common skin conditions, such as acne, eczema, and rashes, can be managed effectively with the help of healing herbs and natural remedies. In this chapter, we will explore various herbs beneficial for skin health, share DIY herbal skincare recipes, and provide a recipe for a soothing Calendula and Aloe Healing Salve to support healthy, radiant skin.

Healing Herbs for Skin Conditions (Acne, Eczema, Rashes)

Natural herbs have been used for centuries to promote skin health and treat various skin ailments. Here are some of the most effective healing herbs for common skin conditions:

1. **Calendula** – Known for its anti-inflammatory, antiseptic, and healing properties, calendula is particularly effective for soothing skin irritations, rashes, and minor burns. Its gentle nature makes it suitable for all skin types, including sensitive skin.

2. **Aloe Vera** – Renowned for its cooling and soothing properties, aloe vera is effective for treating sunburn, acne, and eczema. It hydrates the skin, promotes healing, and has anti-inflammatory effects that calm irritated skin.

3. **Tea Tree Oil** – This powerful essential oil is well-known for its antibacterial and antifungal properties, making it ideal for treating acne and preventing breakouts. It helps reduce inflammation and redness, providing relief for inflamed skin.

4. **Chamomile** – Chamomile's anti-inflammatory and calming effects make it beneficial for a variety of skin issues, including eczema and rosacea. Chamomile can soothe irritation and redness while promoting overall skin healing.

5. **Lavender** – Lavender not only has a calming scent but also provides antiseptic and anti-inflammatory benefits. It's effective for acne, minor burns, and insect bites, and helps promote healing while reducing scarring.

6. **Nettle** – Nettle is rich in vitamins and minerals, making it a fantastic herb for skin health. Its anti-inflammatory properties help treat conditions like eczema and acne, while its high silica content promotes healthy skin and hair.

7. **Witch Hazel** – Known for its astringent properties, witch hazel is excellent for oily and acne-prone skin. It helps tighten pores, reduce inflammation, and soothe irritation, making it an effective natural toner.

DIY Herbal Skincare Recipes

Creating your own herbal skincare products can be rewarding and empowering, allowing you to tailor remedies to your specific skin needs. Here are a few simple DIY recipes for you to try at home:

1. **Calendula Infused Oil**

   o **Ingredients**:

     - 1 cup olive oil or sweet almond oil

     - ½ cup dried calendula petals

   o **Instructions**:

1. Place the dried calendula petals in a clean glass jar.

2. Pour the oil over the petals until they are fully submerged.

3. Seal the jar and place it in a sunny windowsill for 4-6 weeks, shaking it gently every few days.

4. Strain the oil through a fine mesh strainer or cheesecloth and store in a dark glass bottle. Use it as a moisturizer or for creating salves.

2. **Soothing Chamomile Face Mask**

- o **Ingredients**:
  - 2 tbsp dried chamomile flowers
  - 2 tbsp plain yogurt
  - 1 tbsp honey
- o **Instructions**:
  0. Steep the dried chamomile in hot water for 10 minutes, then strain and let cool.
  1. In a bowl, mix the cooled chamomile tea with yogurt and honey to form a paste.
  2. Apply the mask to your face and leave it on for 15-20 minutes, then rinse with warm water. This mask soothes irritated skin and hydrates.

3. **Herbal Facial Toner**

- o **Ingredients**:
  - 1 cup distilled water
  - 1 tbsp dried rose petals
  - 1 tbsp dried lavender
  - 1 tbsp witch hazel
- o **Instructions**:
  0. Boil the distilled water and pour it over the dried rose and lavender in a heatproof jar.
  1. Cover and steep for 30 minutes, then strain out the herbs.
  2. Add witch hazel to the cooled tea and transfer to a spray bottle. Use it as a refreshing facial toner after cleansing.

Recipe: Calendula and Aloe Healing Salve

This nourishing salve combines the healing properties of calendula and aloe vera to soothe and repair damaged skin, making it perfect for minor cuts, rashes, or dry patches.

Ingredients:

- ½ cup calendula-infused oil (from the earlier recipe)

- ¼ cup coconut oil

- ¼ cup beeswax (grated or pastilles)

- 2 tbsp fresh aloe vera gel (or 1 tbsp dried aloe powder)

- Optional: 10-15 drops of lavender essential oil (for added fragrance and benefits)

Instructions:

1. **Melt the Base**: In a double boiler, combine the calendula-infused oil, coconut oil, and beeswax. Heat gently until everything is melted and well combined.

2. **Add Aloe**: Remove from heat and let it cool slightly. Add the fresh aloe vera gel or dried aloe powder and stir well to incorporate. If using, add lavender essential oil and mix thoroughly.

3. **Pour and Set**: Pour the mixture into clean, sterilized containers (small jars or tins). Let the salve cool and set completely at room temperature.

4. **Store**: Label the containers and store them in a cool, dark place. The salve should last for several months.

Usage:

- Apply a small amount of the salve to affected areas as needed, whether for dry patches, rashes, or minor cuts. The combination of calendula and aloe works synergistically to promote healing and soothe inflammation.

Herbs have long been valued for their healing properties and can play a significant role in maintaining healthy skin and promoting natural beauty. By incorporating healing herbs like calendula, aloe vera, and chamomile into your skincare routine, you can treat various skin conditions while enhancing your overall skin health. With simple DIY recipes, you can create effective, natural skincare products tailored to your unique needs, empowering you to embrace your skin's natural beauty.

Chapter 9

Hormonal Balance and Reproductive Health

Hormonal balance plays a crucial role in overall health, influencing everything from mood and energy levels to reproductive function. Many women experience hormonal fluctuations throughout their lives, especially during menstruation and menopause. Fortunately, numerous herbs can help alleviate symptoms related to hormonal imbalances and support reproductive health. In this chapter, we will explore key herbs for menstrual relief and menopause support, natural solutions for fertility, and provide a recipe for Raspberry Leaf Tea, which is particularly beneficial for women's health.

Herbs for Menstrual Relief and Menopause Support

Herbs have been used for centuries to manage menstrual discomfort and support women through various stages of life, including menopause. Here are some powerful herbs that can provide relief from menstrual symptoms and assist with menopause:

1. **Chaste Tree (Vitex)** – Chaste tree is a renowned herb for balancing hormones. It can help alleviate symptoms of premenstrual syndrome (PMS), such as mood swings and breast tenderness, by influencing the pituitary gland's regulation of progesterone.

2. **Cramp Bark** – As the name suggests, cramp bark is particularly effective for relieving menstrual cramps and spasms. It helps relax the smooth muscles of the uterus, providing relief from pain during menstruation.

3. **Dong Quai** – Often referred to as the "female ginseng," dong quai has been traditionally used in Chinese medicine to support women's reproductive health. It can help alleviate menstrual pain and regulate menstrual cycles, making it beneficial for those with irregular periods.

4. **Black Cohosh** – This herb is well-known for its ability to support women during menopause. Black cohosh can help alleviate hot flashes, night sweats, and mood swings associated with hormonal changes during this stage of life.

5. **Red Clover** – Rich in phytoestrogens, red clover can help alleviate symptoms of menopause, such as hot flashes and mood changes. It may also support menstrual health and regularity.

6. **Fennel** – Fennel seeds are often used to relieve bloating and cramping associated with menstruation. They have mild estrogenic properties, which can help balance hormones and ease menstrual discomfort.

Natural Solutions for Fertility and Reproductive Wellness

Many women seek natural ways to enhance fertility and support reproductive health. Several herbs can help regulate hormonal balance and improve reproductive function, making them valuable allies on the journey to conception:

1. **Maca Root** – This adaptogenic herb is known for its ability to support hormonal balance and enhance fertility. Maca can improve libido, regulate menstrual cycles, and boost overall energy levels.

2. **Nettle Leaf** – Nettle is nutrient-rich and supports overall reproductive health. Its high vitamin and mineral content, including iron and folate, makes it beneficial for women trying to conceive.

3. **Red Raspberry Leaf** – Often called the "woman's herb," red raspberry leaf is known for its ability to tone the uterus, support menstrual health, and enhance fertility. It is particularly beneficial in the second half of the menstrual cycle.

4. **Ashwagandha** – Another adaptogen, ashwagandha helps the body cope with stress and supports hormonal balance. It can improve reproductive health by enhancing ovarian function and regulating menstrual cycles.

5. **Evening Primrose Oil** – This oil is rich in gamma-linolenic acid (GLA), which can help improve cervical mucus and support hormonal balance, making it helpful for women trying to conceive.

6. **Ginseng** – Korean ginseng is believed to improve reproductive function and increase libido. It supports hormonal balance and may help regulate the menstrual cycle.

Recipe: Raspberry Leaf Tea for Women's Health

Raspberry leaf tea is a traditional herbal remedy that has been used for centuries to support women's health. It is especially beneficial for menstrual health, pregnancy, and postpartum recovery. The tea is rich in vitamins and minerals, particularly vitamins A, C, and E, as well as calcium, magnesium, and iron.

Ingredients:

- 1-2 teaspoons dried raspberry leaves (or 1 teabag)

- 1 cup boiling water

- Honey or lemon (optional, for flavor)

Instructions:

1. **Steep the Tea**: Place the dried raspberry leaves in a teapot or cup. Pour boiling water over the leaves and cover to steep for 10-15 minutes.

2. **Strain**: After steeping, strain the leaves using a fine mesh strainer or remove the teabag.

3. **Serve**: Add honey or lemon to taste, if desired, and enjoy your tea warm.

Usage:

- Drink 1-2 cups of raspberry leaf tea daily, particularly in the days leading up to your menstrual cycle or during pregnancy. It is also excellent for postpartum recovery.

Hormonal balance is essential for women's health and well-being. By incorporating these healing herbs into your daily routine, you can support menstrual health, manage menopausal symptoms, and enhance fertility naturally. Whether you choose to drink raspberry leaf tea, take herbal supplements, or create your own herbal blends, nature provides a wealth of options to help you nurture your body and promote reproductive wellness. By embracing these natural remedies, you empower yourself to take control of your health and well-being throughout all stages of life.

Chapter 10

Respiratory Health and Allergies

Respiratory health is vital for overall well-being, as our respiratory system is responsible for delivering oxygen to our bodies and removing carbon dioxide. Many people suffer from respiratory issues, including asthma, allergies, and bronchitis, which can significantly impact daily life. Fortunately, herbal remedies can provide natural support and relief for these conditions. In this chapter, we will explore herbal remedies for respiratory issues, discuss natural methods for easing allergies, and share a recipe for an Herbal Steam for Sinus Relief.

Herbal Remedies for Respiratory Issues (Asthma, Allergies, Bronchitis)

Herbs can play a crucial role in supporting respiratory health and managing symptoms of various respiratory conditions. Here are some effective herbs for addressing asthma, allergies, and bronchitis:

1. **Thyme** – Thyme is a powerful antimicrobial and antispasmodic herb that can help soothe respiratory issues, including bronchitis. It acts as an expectorant, helping to loosen mucus in the airways, making it easier to cough up.

2. **Mullein** – Mullein leaves have been used traditionally to treat respiratory ailments. It acts as a soothing demulcent and expectorant, making it effective for easing coughs and promoting lung health. Mullein tea or tincture can help relieve bronchial irritation.

3. **Licorice Root** – Licorice root has anti-inflammatory properties that can help soothe the throat and reduce irritation in the respiratory tract. It's often used to relieve coughs and is beneficial for those with bronchitis or asthma.

4. **Eucalyptus** – Eucalyptus oil is known for its decongestant properties, making it beneficial for respiratory conditions. Inhalation of eucalyptus steam can help clear

nasal passages and ease coughs, while topical application can provide relief from muscle tension and inflammation.

5. **Peppermint** – The menthol in peppermint has a soothing effect on the throat and acts as a natural decongestant. It can help relieve coughs, sinus congestion, and asthma symptoms. Peppermint tea or inhaling peppermint steam can provide quick relief.

6. **Coltsfoot** – Coltsfoot is traditionally used for respiratory issues due to its soothing properties. It can help calm coughs and support lung health by reducing inflammation and irritation.

7. **Nettle** – Nettle is a natural antihistamine and can help reduce allergy symptoms, making it effective for hay fever and other allergic reactions. It's often consumed as a tea or in capsule form.

Easing Allergies Naturally

Allergies can be frustrating and debilitating, but there are several natural methods to ease symptoms:

1. **Quercetin** – A natural flavonoid found in foods like apples, onions, and citrus fruits, quercetin can help stabilize mast cells and reduce histamine release, thereby alleviating allergy symptoms. It is available in supplement form or can be increased in your diet.

2. **Local Honey** – Consuming local honey may help reduce pollen allergies over time. The theory is that small amounts of local pollen in the honey can act like a natural vaccine, helping your body build resistance.

3. **Butterbur** – This herb has shown promise in reducing the severity of allergic rhinitis symptoms. It acts similarly to antihistamines but without the drowsiness often associated with conventional allergy medications.

4. **Probiotics** – Maintaining gut health can support a robust immune system and help alleviate allergy symptoms. Fermented foods like yogurt, kefir, and sauerkraut, or probiotic supplements can be beneficial.

5. **Saline Nasal Rinse** – Rinsing your nasal passages with a saline solution can help remove allergens, mucus, and irritants from the nasal cavity, providing relief from congestion and sneezing.

Recipe: Herbal Steam for Sinus Relief

Herbal steam inhalation is an effective way to relieve sinus congestion and support respiratory health. This recipe combines several beneficial herbs to create a soothing steam for sinus relief.

Ingredients:

- 1 tablespoon dried eucalyptus leaves

- 1 tablespoon dried peppermint leaves

- 1 tablespoon dried thyme leaves

- 1 tablespoon dried chamomile flowers

- 4 cups boiling water

- Optional: 1-2 drops of eucalyptus or peppermint essential oil

Instructions:

1. **Prepare the Herbs**: In a large bowl, combine the dried eucalyptus, peppermint, thyme, and chamomile.

2. **Boil Water**: Bring 4 cups of water to a rolling boil.

3. **Combine**: Carefully pour the boiling water over the herbal mixture in the bowl.

4. **Create a Steam Tent**: Lean over the bowl, keeping your face about 12 inches away from the hot water. Drape a towel over your head and the bowl to trap the steam. Make sure to take breaks as needed to avoid discomfort.

5. **Inhale the Steam**: Close your eyes and inhale the steam deeply for 5-10 minutes. If using, add 1-2 drops of essential oil to the water for an added boost.

6. **Aftercare**: After steaming, drink a glass of water to stay hydrated. You may also want to follow up with a saline nasal rinse to clear out any remaining mucus.

Herbs and natural remedies offer a wealth of options for supporting respiratory health and alleviating symptoms of allergies and respiratory conditions. By incorporating herbs like thyme, mullein, and eucalyptus into your routine, you can naturally enhance your respiratory function and find relief from discomfort. With the addition of simple practices like herbal steam inhalation and dietary adjustments, you can empower yourself to manage respiratory health holistically. Embracing these natural approaches fosters not only physical wellness but also a deeper connection to the healing power of plants.

Chapter 11

Heart Health and Circulation

Heart health is paramount to overall well-being, as the heart and circulatory system play critical roles in supplying oxygen and nutrients to the body. Maintaining a healthy heart can prevent cardiovascular diseases, high blood pressure, and cholesterol issues. This chapter will explore various herbs that promote heart health, support circulation, and enhance cardiovascular function. Additionally, we will provide a recipe for a Hawthorn Berry Tincture, renowned for its heart-supporting properties.

Herbs for Heart Health, Blood Pressure, and Cholesterol

Several herbs have been identified as beneficial for promoting heart health and managing blood pressure and cholesterol levels. Here are some of the most effective:

1. **Hawthorn** – Hawthorn is well-known for its heart-strengthening properties. It helps improve blood flow, lower blood pressure, and reduce symptoms of heart failure. Its berries, leaves, and flowers contain antioxidants that protect the heart from oxidative stress.

2. **Garlic** – Garlic has long been praised for its cardiovascular benefits. It can help lower blood pressure, reduce cholesterol levels, and improve circulation. The active compound allicin is responsible for many of garlic's health benefits.

3. **Ginger** – Ginger is known for its anti-inflammatory properties, which can benefit heart health. It can help improve circulation, lower cholesterol levels, and reduce blood pressure. Additionally, ginger can aid digestion and enhance overall wellness.

4. **Turmeric** – The active ingredient in turmeric, curcumin, has powerful anti-inflammatory and antioxidant effects. It may help reduce inflammation in the cardiovascular system, improve endothelial function, and lower cholesterol levels.

5. **Cayenne Pepper** – Cayenne contains capsaicin, which may help improve circulation and support healthy blood pressure levels. It acts as a natural blood thinner, helping to prevent blood clots and improve overall cardiovascular health.

6. **Milk Thistle** – While primarily known for its liver-supporting properties, milk thistle can also have positive effects on heart health. It helps reduce cholesterol levels and has antioxidant properties that protect the heart.

7. **Green Tea** – Rich in catechins, green tea has been shown to support heart health by lowering LDL cholesterol and improving blood vessel function. Regular consumption can also aid in maintaining a healthy weight.

Supporting Circulation and Cardiovascular Function

Maintaining healthy circulation is essential for optimal heart function and overall health. In addition to herbal remedies, several lifestyle practices can support circulation and cardiovascular function:

1. **Regular Exercise** – Physical activity strengthens the heart, improves circulation, and helps maintain healthy blood pressure and cholesterol levels. Aim for at least 150 minutes of moderate aerobic activity per week.

2. **Balanced Diet** – A heart-healthy diet rich in fruits, vegetables, whole grains, lean proteins, and healthy fats can support cardiovascular health. Foods high in omega-3 fatty acids, such as fatty fish, walnuts, and flaxseeds, are particularly beneficial.

3. **Hydration** – Staying well-hydrated helps maintain blood volume and circulation. Aim to drink plenty of water throughout the day, especially during physical activity.

4. **Stress Management** – Chronic stress can negatively impact heart health. Incorporating stress-reducing practices such as yoga, meditation, and deep-breathing exercises can support cardiovascular function.

5. **Avoiding Tobacco and Limiting Alcohol** – Smoking and excessive alcohol consumption can contribute to cardiovascular problems. Quitting smoking and limiting alcohol intake can significantly improve heart health.

Recipe: Hawthorn Berry Tincture for Heart Health

Hawthorn berries are a potent remedy for supporting heart health and improving circulation. Making a tincture allows for the concentrated extraction of the beneficial compounds found in hawthorn berries, making it easy to incorporate into your daily routine.

Ingredients:

- 1 cup dried hawthorn berries (or 1.5 cups fresh berries)

- 2 cups high-proof alcohol (such as vodka or brandy)

- Optional: 1 teaspoon dried hawthorn leaves or flowers for additional benefits

Instructions:

1. **Prepare the Jar**: In a clean glass jar, combine the dried hawthorn berries (and leaves or flowers, if using).

2. **Add Alcohol**: Pour the high-proof alcohol over the hawthorn berries until they are completely submerged. Leave a little space at the top of the jar.

3. **Seal and Shake**: Seal the jar tightly and shake it gently to mix the ingredients.

4. **Infusion Period**: Place the jar in a cool, dark place for 4-6 weeks. Shake the jar gently every few days to help the extraction process.

5. **Strain**: After 4-6 weeks, strain the mixture through a fine mesh strainer or cheesecloth into a clean glass bottle. Be sure to squeeze out any excess liquid from the hawthorn berries.

6. **Label and Store**: Label the bottle with the date and store it in a cool, dark place. The tincture should last for several years.

Dosage:

- Take 1-2 droppers full of the hawthorn berry tincture 1-3 times daily, or as recommended by a healthcare professional. You can take it directly or mix it into water or herbal tea.

Heart health is a vital aspect of overall wellness, and nature provides a wealth of herbal remedies to support cardiovascular function and circulation. Incorporating herbs like hawthorn, garlic, and ginger into your daily routine can help maintain a healthy heart and manage blood pressure and cholesterol levels. Additionally, adopting heart-healthy lifestyle practices can further enhance your cardiovascular health. By taking proactive steps to care for your heart, you empower yourself to live a vibrant, healthy life. Embrace the power of plants and the wisdom of natural remedies as you nurture your heart and overall well-being.

Chapter 12

Energy and Vitality Boosters

In our fast-paced world, maintaining energy and vitality is essential for productivity and overall well-being. Many people struggle with fatigue, stress, and mental fog, making it crucial to explore natural solutions that can enhance daily energy levels and resilience. This chapter will delve into herbal tonics that promote energy and endurance, highlight adaptogens that support stress resilience and mental clarity, and provide a delicious recipe for an Ashwagandha and Maca Energy Elixir.

Herbal Tonics for Daily Energy and Endurance

Herbal tonics can serve as powerful allies in boosting energy levels and enhancing physical endurance. Here are some herbs renowned for their energizing properties:

1. **Ginseng** – One of the most well-known adaptogenic herbs, ginseng is celebrated for its ability to enhance energy levels, reduce fatigue, and improve physical performance. Both Asian (Panax) and American ginseng have unique properties that can support vitality.

2. **Rhodiola Rosea** – Rhodiola is an adaptogen that helps the body adapt to stress and can improve stamina and energy levels. It is particularly beneficial for enhancing physical performance and reducing fatigue during intense exercise.

3. **Eleuthero (Siberian Ginseng)** – Eleuthero is often used to combat fatigue and enhance endurance. It may improve mental clarity and physical performance, making it an excellent choice for athletes and anyone needing a boost.

4. **Cordyceps** – This medicinal mushroom has been traditionally used to increase energy and endurance. Cordyceps can enhance oxygen utilization in the body, making it a favorite among athletes for improved performance.

5. **Green Tea** – Besides being rich in antioxidants, green tea contains caffeine and L-theanine, which together provide a balanced energy boost without the jitters associated with other caffeinated drinks. It's an excellent choice for maintaining alertness throughout the day.

6. **Beetroot** – Beetroot is a natural source of nitrates, which can improve blood flow and oxygen delivery to muscles. Drinking beetroot juice before exercise can enhance endurance and boost energy levels.

Adaptogens for Stress Resilience and Mental Clarity

Adaptogens are herbs that help the body adapt to stress, promote balance, and enhance mental clarity. Incorporating adaptogens into your daily routine can significantly impact energy levels and cognitive function. Here are some powerful adaptogens to consider:

1. **Ashwagandha** – Known for its ability to reduce stress and anxiety, ashwagandha also boosts energy levels and improves mental clarity. It can enhance stamina and endurance, making it an excellent choice for busy individuals.

2. **Holy Basil (Tulsi)** – Holy basil is revered for its calming effects and ability to enhance mental clarity. It helps reduce stress and anxiety while boosting energy levels, making it a fantastic adaptogen for everyday wellness.

3. **Maca Root** – Maca is known for its energizing properties and ability to enhance stamina and endurance. It is also recognized for balancing hormones and improving mood, making it beneficial for overall vitality.

4. **Gotu Kola** – This herb is known for its cognitive-enhancing properties, promoting mental clarity and focus. Gotu kola is often used to support memory and concentration, making it an excellent addition for those seeking to boost productivity.

5. **Schisandra** – Schisandra berries are known for their adaptogenic properties and ability to enhance physical performance and mental clarity. They can help the body cope with stress while promoting energy and endurance.

Recipe: Ashwagandha and Maca Energy Elixir

This delightful energy elixir combines the energizing properties of ashwagandha and maca with other nutritious ingredients to create a revitalizing drink that supports energy, vitality, and stress resilience.

Ingredients:

- 1 teaspoon ashwagandha powder

- 1 teaspoon maca powder

- 1 tablespoon honey or maple syrup (adjust for sweetness)

- 1 cup milk (or plant-based milk of choice, such as almond, oat, or coconut milk)

- 1/2 teaspoon vanilla extract (optional)

- A pinch of cinnamon (optional)

- Ice (optional, for a chilled drink)

Instructions:

1. **Heat the Milk**: In a small saucepan, gently heat the milk over medium heat until warm (but not boiling). If you prefer a chilled elixir, skip this step.

2. **Mix the Ingredients**: In a separate bowl or blender, combine the ashwagandha powder, maca powder, honey or maple syrup, vanilla extract, and cinnamon. Add a splash of the warm milk to create a smooth paste.

3. **Combine**: Slowly whisk the paste into the warm milk until fully incorporated. If using a blender, blend on low until smooth and frothy.

4. **Serve**: Pour the elixir into a glass. If desired, serve over ice for a refreshing drink.

5. **Enjoy**: Sip and enjoy this nourishing energy elixir as a mid-morning or afternoon pick-me-up!

Incorporating herbal tonics and adaptogens into your daily routine can significantly enhance energy levels, improve endurance, and promote mental clarity. By embracing nature's powerful remedies like ginseng, ashwagandha, and maca, you can foster resilience against stress and fatigue. This holistic approach not only supports your physical well-being but also nurtures your mental and emotional health. By prioritizing energy and vitality through herbal remedies, you empower yourself to lead a vibrant, fulfilling life. Embrace these natural solutions and thrive in your everyday wellness journey!

Chapter 13

Building a Strong Immune Defense System

A robust immune system is essential for maintaining health and wellness throughout the year. It protects the body against infections, viruses, and diseases, playing a crucial role in our overall well-being. This chapter will explore strategies for strengthening immunity year-round, herbal approaches for flu season and beyond, and a delicious recipe for Fire Cider, a traditional tonic known for its immune-boosting properties.

Strengthening Immunity Year-Round

To support a strong immune system, it's important to adopt a holistic approach that includes lifestyle choices, dietary habits, and stress management. Here are several key strategies to enhance immunity throughout the year:

1. **Balanced Nutrition**: Consuming a diet rich in fruits, vegetables, whole grains, lean proteins, and healthy fats provides essential vitamins and minerals that support immune function. Key nutrients include:

   o **Vitamin C:** Found in citrus fruits, bell peppers, and broccoli, it helps stimulate the production of white blood cells.

   o **Vitamin D:** Important for immune regulation, vitamin D can be obtained from sunlight, fatty fish, fortified foods, and supplements.

   o **Zinc:** Essential for immune cell development, zinc is found in nuts, seeds, legumes, and whole grains.

2. **Regular Exercise**: Physical activity improves circulation and promotes the efficient functioning of immune cells. Aim for at least 150 minutes of moderate aerobic activity each week to maintain a strong immune system.

3. **Adequate Sleep**: Quality sleep is crucial for immune health. Aim for 7-9 hours of restful sleep each night to help the body recover and rejuvenate.

4. **Hydration**: Staying well-hydrated helps support overall bodily functions, including the immune system. Aim to drink plenty of water throughout the day.

5. **Stress Management**: Chronic stress can weaken the immune system. Incorporating stress-reduction techniques such as meditation, yoga, and deep-breathing exercises can support immune health.

6. **Avoiding Tobacco and Limiting Alcohol**: Smoking and excessive alcohol consumption can impair immune function. Quitting smoking and moderating alcohol intake can greatly enhance overall health.

Herbal Strategies for Flu Season and Beyond

Herbs have long been used to bolster the immune system and provide support during flu season. Here are some effective herbal strategies:

1. **Elderberry** – Elderberry is well-known for its antiviral properties and can help reduce the duration and severity of flu symptoms. Elderberry syrup is a popular remedy for immune support during cold and flu season.

2. **Echinacea** – Often used at the onset of illness, echinacea can help stimulate the immune response and reduce the duration of colds and flu. It's available in various forms, including teas, tinctures, and capsules.

3. **Astragalus** – This adaptogenic herb is known for its immune-boosting properties. Astragalus root can help protect against infections and enhance the body's overall resilience.

4. **Ginger** – Ginger has anti-inflammatory and antimicrobial properties, making it beneficial for fighting infections and supporting digestive health, which is closely linked to immune function.

5. **Turmeric** – With its potent anti-inflammatory and antioxidant properties, turmeric can support immune health and help the body combat inflammation.

6. **Oregano Oil** – Known for its antimicrobial properties, oregano oil can help fight infections. It's often used as a natural remedy for respiratory issues and other infections.

Recipe: Fire Cider for Immune Support

Fire Cider is a traditional herbal tonic made from a blend of powerful ingredients known for their immune-boosting properties. This spicy, tangy elixir is easy to make and can be taken daily to support overall health.

Ingredients:

- 1 cup apple cider vinegar (raw, unfiltered)
- 1 onion, chopped
- 10 cloves garlic, minced
- 1-2 tablespoons ginger, grated
- 1-2 tablespoons horseradish, grated (optional for added heat)
- 1-2 fresh jalapeños or chili peppers, sliced (adjust to taste)
- 1 tablespoon turmeric powder or fresh turmeric, grated
- 1 tablespoon honey (adjust for sweetness)
- Optional: Additional herbs such as rosemary, thyme, or oregano for flavor

Instructions:

1. **Combine Ingredients**: In a quart-sized mason jar, combine the chopped onion, minced garlic, grated ginger, horseradish (if using), sliced jalapeños, turmeric, and any optional herbs.

2. **Add Vinegar**: Pour the apple cider vinegar over the herbs until the jar is full. Seal the jar tightly with a lid.

3. **Infusion Period**: Place the jar in a cool, dark place for at least 2-4 weeks. Shake the jar daily to help infuse the flavors and benefits of the ingredients.

4. **Strain and Sweeten**: After 2-4 weeks, strain the mixture through a fine mesh strainer or cheesecloth into a clean glass jar. Press down to extract as much liquid as possible. Stir in honey to taste.

5. **Store**: Store the Fire Cider in the refrigerator for up to a year.

How to Use:

- Take 1-2 tablespoons of Fire Cider daily as a preventive measure during cold and flu season. You can take it straight, mix it into warm water, or add it to salad dressings for a zesty kick.

Building a strong immune defense system requires a multifaceted approach that includes healthy lifestyle choices, proper nutrition, and the use of herbal remedies. By integrating strategies such as maintaining a balanced diet, exercising regularly, managing stress, and utilizing herbs like elderberry and echinacea, you can significantly enhance your body's natural defenses against illness. With the addition of powerful tonics like Fire Cider, you can support your immune health and navigate cold and flu season with confidence. Embrace these natural solutions to empower your immune system and promote long-lasting health and vitality.

Chapter 14

Detox and Cleansing with Herbs

Detoxification is a vital process that helps the body eliminate toxins and maintain overall health. While the body has its natural detoxification mechanisms, such as the liver, kidneys, and digestive system, incorporating herbal remedies can enhance these processes. This chapter will explore how to support these organs, introduce gentle cleansing herbs, and provide a nourishing recipe for Dandelion and Burdock Root Detox Tea.

Supporting the Liver, Kidneys, and Digestive Tract

The liver, kidneys, and digestive tract are essential organs in the body's detoxification system. Supporting their health can improve the body's ability to eliminate toxins effectively. Here are some ways to support each of these vital organs:

1. **Liver Support**: The liver is the primary organ for detoxification, processing nutrients and filtering toxins from the bloodstream. To support liver health:

   - **Hydration**: Drink plenty of water to help the liver flush out toxins.

   - **Healthy Diet**: Incorporate foods rich in antioxidants and healthy fats, such as leafy greens, cruciferous vegetables, avocados, and nuts.

   - **Herbs**: Milk thistle, dandelion root, and artichoke are excellent herbs for liver support, known for their ability to promote liver function and protect against damage.

2. **Kidney Support**: The kidneys filter waste and excess fluids from the blood. To support kidney health:

   - **Hydration**: Staying well-hydrated is crucial for kidney function and helps prevent the formation of kidney stones.

   - **Balanced Diet**: Focus on a diet low in sodium and high in fruits and vegetables to support kidney health.

- **Herbs**: Nettle leaf, parsley, and marshmallow root can promote kidney health by supporting urinary function and reducing inflammation.

3. **Digestive Tract Support**: A healthy digestive tract is essential for proper detoxification. To support digestive health:

   - **Fiber-Rich Foods**: Incorporate fiber from fruits, vegetables, and whole grains to promote regular bowel movements and eliminate waste.

   - **Probiotics**: Include fermented foods such as yogurt, sauerkraut, and kefir to support gut health and improve digestion.

   - **Herbs**: Ginger, peppermint, and fennel can aid digestion and help relieve bloating and discomfort.

Gentle Cleansing Herbs for a Healthy System

Gentle cleansing herbs can help the body detoxify without harsh side effects. Here are some effective herbs for promoting detoxification:

1. **Dandelion** – Dandelion root and leaves are excellent for supporting liver function and promoting bile production. They can also act as a diuretic, helping to eliminate excess fluid from the body.

2. **Burdock Root** – Burdock root is known for its blood-purifying properties. It helps detoxify the blood, supports liver function, and aids digestion, making it an excellent herb for cleansing.

3. **Nettle** – Nettle leaf is a natural diuretic that supports kidney function and helps eliminate toxins through urine. It's also rich in vitamins and minerals, making it a nutritious addition to any detox regimen.

4. **Milk Thistle** – The active compound in milk thistle, silymarin, protects the liver from toxins and promotes its regenerative abilities. It's often used in detox programs to support liver health.

5. **Red Clover** – Red clover is traditionally used as a blood purifier. It supports lymphatic function and may help eliminate toxins from the body.

6. **Cilantro** – Cilantro is known for its ability to help remove heavy metals and other toxins from the body. It can be added to salads, smoothies, or soups for an extra detox boost.

This soothing detox tea combines the cleansing properties of dandelion and burdock root, creating a nourishing beverage that supports liver and digestive health.

Ingredients:

- 1 tablespoon dried dandelion root (or 1-2 teaspoons fresh dandelion root, chopped)
- 1 tablespoon dried burdock root (or 1-2 teaspoons fresh burdock root, chopped)
- 4 cups water
- Optional: Honey or lemon to taste

Instructions:

1. **Prepare the Roots**: If using fresh dandelion and burdock root, wash and chop them into smaller pieces. If using dried herbs, measure them out.

2. **Boil Water**: In a saucepan, bring 4 cups of water to a boil.

3. **Add Herbs**: Once the water is boiling, add the dandelion and burdock roots. Reduce the heat and let the mixture simmer for 15-20 minutes.

4. **Strain the Tea**: After simmering, remove the saucepan from heat and strain the tea through a fine mesh strainer or cheesecloth into a teapot or pitcher.

5. **Sweeten (Optional)**: Add honey or lemon to taste, if desired.

6. **Serve**: Enjoy the tea warm, or let it cool and serve over ice for a refreshing iced detox tea.

Note: Drink this detox tea 1-2 times daily, especially during a detox regimen, to support your body's natural cleansing processes.

Detoxification is an essential aspect of maintaining health and vitality. By supporting the liver, kidneys, and digestive tract, you can enhance your body's ability to eliminate toxins effectively. Incorporating gentle cleansing herbs like dandelion and burdock root can promote overall wellness and vitality. Enjoying nourishing herbal teas, along with healthy lifestyle choices, empowers you to embrace detoxification as a path to optimal health. As you integrate these practices into your routine, you will foster a healthier, more vibrant you, ready to face each day with renewed energy and clarity.

Chapter 15

Herbs for Mental Clarity and Focus

In our increasingly fast-paced world, mental clarity and focus are crucial for productivity, learning, and overall cognitive health. Certain herbs, known as nootropics, can enhance brain function, improve memory, and boost cognitive performance. This chapter will explore effective nootropic herbs for brain health, provide tips for improving focus and cognitive function, and share a delicious recipe for a Rosemary and Ginkgo Memory Booster.

Nootropic Herbs for Brain Health and Memory

Nootropic herbs have been used for centuries in various cultures to enhance cognitive function and support brain health. Here are some of the most effective nootropic herbs:

1. **Ginkgo Biloba**: Known for its ability to improve blood circulation to the brain, Ginkgo Biloba is often used to enhance memory and cognitive function. It may also help with symptoms of anxiety and depression.

2. **Rosemary**: Traditionally associated with memory improvement, rosemary has antioxidant properties that can protect brain cells from damage. Its aroma has been shown to enhance concentration and memory recall.

3. **Bacopa Monnieri**: This herb is renowned for its cognitive-enhancing properties. Bacopa is believed to improve memory, reduce anxiety, and support overall brain health by promoting synaptic communication.

4. **Rhodiola Rosea**: An adaptogen known for its ability to combat fatigue and stress, Rhodiola also has neuroprotective properties that can enhance cognitive performance, particularly in stressful situations.

5. **Panax Ginseng**: This powerful adaptogen is believed to enhance cognitive performance, improve attention, and reduce mental fatigue. It may also support memory and overall brain health.

6. **Lion's Mane Mushroom**: This medicinal mushroom is known for its neuroprotective properties and ability to stimulate the production of nerve growth factor (NGF), which is essential for the growth and maintenance of neurons.

7. **Ashwagandha**: Known primarily for its stress-reducing properties, ashwagandha may also support cognitive function and memory by reducing cortisol levels and promoting a sense of calm.

8. **Gotu Kola**: This herb is often used to improve mental clarity and concentration. It is believed to enhance cognitive function, memory, and learning ability.

Recipes and Tips for Improved Focus and Cognitive Function

Incorporating nootropic herbs into your daily routine can significantly enhance mental clarity and focus. Here are some practical tips and recipes to help you boost cognitive function:

1. **Herbal Teas**: Make a blend of nootropic herbs such as rosemary, ginkgo, and peppermint. Steep in hot water for 5-10 minutes for a refreshing and focus-enhancing tea.

2. **Smoothie Boosters**: Add powdered forms of nootropic herbs like Bacopa or Lion's Mane to your morning smoothie for an easy and nutritious way to support brain health.

3. **Mindful Eating**: Include brain-boosting foods in your diet, such as fatty fish (rich in omega-3 fatty acids), blueberries (antioxidant-rich), and dark chocolate (contains flavonoids). Combine these with nootropic herbs for enhanced benefits.

4. **Hydration**: Stay well-hydrated, as even mild dehydration can impair cognitive function. Infuse your water with lemon, cucumber, or herbs like mint and rosemary for a refreshing drink that supports focus.

5. **Breathing Exercises**: Incorporate mindfulness and deep-breathing exercises into your daily routine. These practices can help reduce stress and enhance focus, allowing your brain to function at its best.

Recipe: Rosemary and Ginkgo Memory Booster

This invigorating beverage combines the cognitive-enhancing properties of rosemary and Ginkgo Biloba with other nutritious ingredients to create a delicious memory-boosting drink.

Ingredients:

- 1 teaspoon dried rosemary (or 1 tablespoon fresh rosemary, chopped)

- 1 teaspoon dried Ginkgo Biloba leaves (or Ginkgo Biloba extract, adjust dosage according to instructions)

- 2 cups water

- 1 tablespoon honey or maple syrup (adjust for sweetness)

- Juice of 1 lemon (optional)

- Ice (optional, for a refreshing drink)

Instructions:

1. **Boil Water**: In a saucepan, bring 2 cups of water to a boil.

2. **Add Herbs**: Once boiling, add the dried rosemary and Ginkgo Biloba leaves to the water. Reduce heat and let the mixture simmer for about 10 minutes.

3. **Strain the Tea**: After simmering, remove from heat and strain the liquid into a glass or teapot using a fine mesh strainer.

4. **Sweeten (Optional)**: Stir in honey or maple syrup to taste. You can also add lemon juice for a refreshing twist.

5. **Serve**: Enjoy the beverage warm, or let it cool and serve over ice for a refreshing iced memory booster.

Enhancing mental clarity and focus through the use of nootropic herbs is a powerful way to support cognitive health and overall well-being. By incorporating herbs like Ginkgo Biloba and rosemary into your daily routine, along with healthy lifestyle practices such as mindful eating, hydration, and stress management, you can foster a sharper, more focused mind. Embrace these natural solutions to boost your cognitive function and memory, enabling you to tackle daily challenges with clarity and confidence. As you explore the benefits of herbal remedies, you empower yourself to unlock your full mental potential.

Chapter 16

Supporting Long-Term Health with Herbs

As we age, maintaining health and vitality becomes increasingly important. Herbs can play a vital role in supporting longevity and promoting graceful aging. This chapter will explore herbs for longevity, herbal supplements for bone and joint health, and a rejuvenating recipe for an Anti-Aging Herbal Tonic.

Herbs for Longevity and Aging Gracefully

Certain herbs have been shown to support long-term health and promote a graceful aging process. Here are some key herbs associated with longevity:

1. **Turmeric**: Curcumin, the active compound in turmeric, has powerful anti-inflammatory and antioxidant properties. It supports joint health, cardiovascular health, and brain function, making it a great ally for aging gracefully.

2. **Ashwagandha**: This adaptogenic herb is known for its ability to reduce stress and promote overall well-being. It may support cognitive health, reduce inflammation, and help maintain energy levels as we age.

3. **Ginseng**: Both Panax ginseng and American ginseng are known for their energizing properties. They support immune function, improve energy levels, and may enhance cognitive function, all of which contribute to healthy aging.

4. **Green Tea**: Rich in antioxidants, particularly catechins, green tea supports cardiovascular health and may protect against chronic diseases. Its anti-Inflammatory properties can also promote healthy skin.

5. **Reishi Mushroom**: Known as the "mushroom of immortality," reishi has immune-boosting and stress-reducing properties. It may enhance overall vitality and support healthy aging.

6. **Holy Basil (Tulsi)**: This adaptogenic herb helps combat stress and promotes emotional well-being. It also has anti-inflammatory and antioxidant properties that support longevity.

7. **Nettle**: Nettle is rich in vitamins and minerals that support overall health. It may help improve joint health, reduce inflammation, and enhance skin vitality.

Herbal Supplements for Bone and Joint Health

Maintaining bone and joint health is crucial as we age. Several herbs can support musculoskeletal health:

1. **Horsetail**: Rich in silica, horsetail is known to strengthen bones and connective tissues. It may help improve bone density and support joint health.

2. **Boswellia**: Boswellia serrata, also known as Indian frankincense, has anti-inflammatory properties that may help relieve joint pain and improve mobility.

3. **Ginger**: Known for its anti-inflammatory properties, ginger can help reduce pain and stiffness in joints. It may be particularly beneficial for those with arthritis.

4. **Willow Bark**: Traditionally used as a natural pain reliever, willow bark contains salicin, which has similar properties to aspirin. It can help relieve pain and inflammation in the joints.

5. **Turmeric**: In addition to its anti-inflammatory benefits, turmeric supports overall joint health and may help prevent the deterioration of cartilage.

6. **Moringa**: Moringa leaves are packed with calcium, magnesium, and other nutrients that support bone health. Its anti-inflammatory properties also contribute to joint health.

Recipe: Anti-Aging Herbal Tonic

This invigorating Anti-Aging Herbal Tonic combines powerful herbs known for their longevity benefits. It's a refreshing drink that supports overall vitality and promotes graceful aging.

Ingredients:

- 1 tablespoon dried turmeric root (or 1 teaspoon turmeric powder)

- 1 teaspoon dried ginger root (or 1/2 teaspoon ginger powder)

- 1 tablespoon dried hibiscus flowers (optional for flavor and color)

- 2 cups water

- 1 tablespoon honey (adjust for sweetness)

- Juice of 1 lemon

- Optional: Fresh mint leaves or basil for garnish

Instructions:

1. **Boil Water**: In a saucepan, bring 2 cups of water to a boil.

2. **Add Ingredients**: Once boiling, add the dried turmeric, ginger, and hibiscus flowers. Reduce heat and let the mixture simmer for about 10-15 minutes.

3. **Strain the Tonic**: After simmering, remove from heat and strain the mixture into a glass or teapot using a fine mesh strainer.

4. **Sweeten and Add Lemon**: Stir in honey to taste and add the juice of one lemon.

5. **Serve**: Enjoy the tonic warm, or let it cool and serve over ice for a refreshing drink. Garnish with fresh mint leaves or basil if desired.

Incorporating herbs into your daily routine can significantly impact long-term health and wellness. By embracing the healing properties of herbs such as turmeric, ashwagandha, and ginseng, you can support longevity and age gracefully. Herbal supplements can also play a vital role in maintaining bone and joint health, ensuring you remain active and vibrant as you age. The Anti-Aging Herbal Tonic is a delicious way to nourish your body and promote vitality. As you cultivate these herbal practices, you empower yourself to lead a healthier, more fulfilling life, celebrating the joys of each stage of aging with grace and strength.

Chapter 17

The Art of Blending Herbs

Herbal blending is both an art and a science, allowing individuals to create personalized remedies that cater to their unique health needs and preferences. This chapter will explore how to effectively combine herbs for maximum therapeutic effect, provide guidance on creating custom blends for personal health goals, and offer a recipe for a Customized Herbal Blend Workbook.

How to Combine Herbs for Maximum Effect

Combining herbs can enhance their effectiveness, as many herbs work synergistically to provide greater health benefits than when taken alone. Here are some key principles for blending herbs effectively:

1. **Understand Herbal Properties**: Before blending, familiarize yourself with the properties of each herb. Consider factors such as flavor profile, primary actions (e.g., anti-inflammatory, relaxing), and possible interactions.

2. **Balance Tastes and Energies**: Aim for a balance of tastes (sweet, bitter, sour, salty, and pungent) and energies (warming, cooling, moistening, and drying) in your blend. This balance can create a more pleasant and effective herbal experience.

3. **Layering Effects**: Combine herbs that target different aspects of the same health concern. For example, if addressing digestive issues, consider combining a soothing herb like peppermint with a digestive stimulant like ginger.

4. **Start Small**: When creating a new blend, start with small quantities of each herb to gauge the taste and effectiveness. Gradually adjust ratios based on personal preferences and desired effects.

5. **Monitor Effects**: Pay attention to how your body responds to the blend. Keep a journal to note any changes in symptoms or feelings, allowing for adjustments to the formula as needed.

Creating Custom Blends for Personal Health Goals

Creating custom herbal blends tailored to your specific health goals can empower you to take control of your wellness journey. Here's a step-by-step approach to developing personalized herbal blends:

1. **Identify Your Health Goals**: Determine what you want to achieve with your blend. Common goals might include stress relief, improved digestion, enhanced energy, or immune support.

2. **Choose Complementary Herbs**: Select herbs that align with your goals. For instance:

   o **Stress Relief**: Consider herbs like chamomile, lemon balm, and ashwagandha.

   o **Digestive Support**: Look at peppermint, ginger, and fennel.

   o **Energy Boost**: Combine ginseng, rhodiola, and green tea.

3. **Determine Ratios**: Decide on the proportions of each herb based on their strengths and your preferences. A common starting point is to use 1 part of the primary herb (the one most associated with your goal) and ½ part each of the supporting herbs.

4. **Prepare Your Blend**: Whether you're making a tea, tincture, or powdered mix, combine your chosen herbs in a clean, dry container. Label the blend with its ingredients and intended purpose.

5. **Test and Adjust**: After using your blend for a week or two, evaluate its effectiveness. Adjust the ratios or add/remove herbs based on your experiences.

Recipe: Customized Herbal Blend Workbook

Creating a Customized Herbal Blend Workbook can help you document your herbal blending journey, track your health goals, and refine your recipes over time. Here's how to create your workbook:

Materials Needed:

- Blank notebook or binder with loose-leaf paper

- Pens or markers

- Dividers (optional)

- Herbal reference books or resources for herb properties and uses.

Workbook Sections:

1. **Herb Profiles:**

   - Create a section for individual herbs. Include the following details:

     - Name of the herb

     - Properties (e.g., medicinal uses, flavor profile)

     - Preparation methods (e.g., tea, tincture, capsules)

     - Dosage guidelines

     - Contraindications and safety considerations

2. **Blend Recipes:**

   - Dedicate pages for your custom blends. Include:

     - Blend name and purpose

     - List of herbs and ratios

     - Preparation method

- Date of creation

- Personal notes on taste and effects

3. **Health Goals**:

   - Create a section to outline your health goals and the blends associated with each. Document progress, challenges, and successes.

4. **Reflection and Adjustment**:

   - Include pages for reflection. After using a blend, note its effectiveness, any side effects, and any adjustments you wish to make for the future.

5. **Resources**:

   - Keep a list of trusted herbal resources, including books, websites, and local herbalists, for further study and inspiration.

The art of blending herbs is a powerful tool for personal wellness, allowing individuals to create customized remedies that address specific health goals. By understanding the properties of various herbs, learning to balance their effects, and documenting your blending experiences in a Customized Herbal Blend Workbook, you can enhance your herbal practice and empower your journey toward optimal health. Embrace the creativity and individuality of herbal blending, and enjoy the process of discovering the perfect combinations for your unique needs.

Instructions:

1. In a saucepan, bring the water to a boil. Add the quinoa, reduce heat, cover, and simmer for 15 minutes or until the water is absorbed. Fluff with a fork and let cool.

2. In a large bowl, combine the cooked quinoa, cherry tomatoes, cucumber, feta, parsley, and basil.

3. In a small bowl, whisk together the olive oil, lemon juice, salt, and pepper. Drizzle over the salad and toss to combine.

4. Serve chilled or at room temperature.

2. Roasted Vegetable Medley with Herbs

Ingredients:

- 2 cups mixed vegetables (e.g., bell peppers, zucchini, carrots, and red onion)

- 2 tablespoons olive oil

- 1 teaspoon dried oregano

- 1 teaspoon dried thyme

- 1 teaspoon garlic powder

- Salt and pepper to taste

Instructions:

1. Preheat the oven to 425°F (220°C).

2. Toss the mixed vegetables in olive oil, oregano, thyme, garlic powder, salt, and pepper until well coated.

3. Spread the vegetables evenly on a baking sheet.

4. Roast for 25-30 minutes, or until the vegetables are tender and slightly caramelized.

5. Serve warm as a side dish.

Recipe: Immune-Boosting Herb-Infused Olive Oil

This herb-infused olive oil combines the immune-boosting properties of various culinary herbs, making it a flavorful addition to salads, pasta, and other dishes.

Ingredients:

- 1 cup extra-virgin olive oil

- 4 cloves garlic, crushed

- 1/4 cup fresh oregano leaves (or 2 tablespoons dried oregano)

- 1/4 cup fresh thyme leaves (or 2 tablespoons dried thyme)

- 1/4 cup fresh basil leaves (or 2 tablespoons dried basil)

- 1/4 teaspoon red pepper flakes (optional, for a kick)

Instructions:

1. In a small saucepan, combine the olive oil, crushed garlic, oregano, thyme, basil, and red pepper flakes (if using).

2. Heat the mixture over low heat for about 15 minutes, allowing the flavors to infuse without boiling.

3. Remove from heat and let cool.

4. Strain the oil through a fine mesh strainer or cheesecloth into a clean, dry bottle, discarding the solids.

5. Seal the bottle and store it in a cool, dark place. Use within a month for the best flavor.

Incorporating culinary herbs into your cooking not only enhances the flavor of your meals but also contributes to your overall health and wellness. By using herbs like basil, oregano, and parsley, you can create delicious dishes that provide medicinal benefits. The Immune-Boosting Herb-Infused Olive Oil is a versatile and flavorful way to elevate your cooking while supporting your immune system. Embrace the art of cooking with herbs, and discover how a herbal lifestyle can lead to improved well-being and enjoyment in your everyday meals.

Chapter 19

Growing and Harvesting Your Own Medicinal Herbs

Growing your own medicinal herbs is a rewarding endeavor that can enhance your herbal practice, provide fresh ingredients for cooking, and offer a deeper connection to the healing properties of plants. This chapter will guide you through the process of starting an herb garden, provide tips for harvesting, drying, and storing herbs, and offer a step-by-step guide to preserving fresh herbs.

How to Start an Herb Garden

Starting your own herb garden can be done in a variety of spaces, from a backyard plot to a few pots on a windowsill. Here's how to get started:

1. Choose the Right Location

- **Sunlight**: Most herbs thrive in full sun, requiring 6-8 hours of direct sunlight each day. Find a sunny spot in your garden or on your balcony.

- **Soil**: Well-draining soil is essential for healthy herbs. You can improve drainage by mixing in compost or sand.

2. Select Your Herbs

Choose a variety of herbs based on your culinary and medicinal interests. Here are some popular choices for beginners:

- **Basil**

- **Oregano**

- **Thyme**

- **Rosemary**

- **Peppermint**

- **Chamomile**

- **Echinacea**

- **Calendula**

3. Decide on Planting Method

- **Seeds**: Start herbs from seeds indoors or directly in the garden, depending on the herb and climate.

- **Transplants**: Purchase young plants from a nursery for quicker results. Look for healthy, robust plants without signs of disease.

4. Planting Your Herbs

- Follow specific planting instructions for each herb regarding depth and spacing.

- Generally, plant seeds or transplants in rows or clusters, ensuring adequate space for growth.

5. Watering and Care

- Water your herbs regularly but avoid overwatering. The soil should be kept moist but not soggy.

- Consider using organic fertilizers to enhance growth, especially during the growing season.

6. Protecting Your Garden

- Monitor for pests and diseases. Use organic pest control methods if necessary, such as insecticidal soap or neem oil.

- Companion planting can help deter pests. For example, planting basil alongside tomatoes can repel aphids.

Tips for Harvesting, Drying, and Storing Herbs

Proper harvesting, drying, and storing of herbs is crucial for preserving their medicinal properties and flavor. Here's how to do it:

1. Harvesting Herbs

- **Timing**: The best time to harvest is in the morning after the dew has dried but before the sun gets too hot. This preserves the essential oils in the herbs.

- **Technique**: Use sharp scissors or pruning shears to cut stems just above a leaf node. This encourages new growth. For leafy herbs, such as basil or parsley, trim leaves from the top of the plant.

2. Drying Herbs

Drying herbs is an effective way to preserve their potency. Here are a few methods:

- **Air Drying**: Bundle stems together and hang them upside down in a cool, dark, and dry place with good airflow. This method can take several days to weeks, depending on humidity.

- **Dehydrator**: Use a food dehydrator set to a low temperature (95-115°F or 35-46°C). Arrange herbs in a single layer and dry until crispy.

- **Oven Drying**: Place herbs on a baking sheet in the oven at the lowest setting (around 180°F or 82°C). Keep the door slightly ajar to allow moisture to escape, and check frequently.

3. Storing Dried Herbs

- Once dried, store herbs in airtight containers away from light, heat, and moisture. Glass jars or dark-colored containers are ideal.

- Label containers with the herb name and date of drying. Most dried herbs retain their potency for 1-3 years, depending on the type.

Step-by-Step Guide to Preserving Fresh Herbs

If you want to preserve the freshness of your herbs rather than drying them, here are some effective methods:

1. Freezing Fresh Herbs

- **Chop and Freeze**: Finely chop your fresh herbs and place them in ice cube trays. Fill the trays with water or olive oil and freeze. Once frozen, transfer the cubes to a labeled zip-top bag for later use in cooking.

- **Whole Leaf Freezing**: Place whole leaves on a baking sheet and freeze until solid. Transfer to a zip-top bag for storage. This method works well for larger leaves like basil and mint.

2. Making Herb Pastes

- Combine fresh herbs with a bit of olive oil in a food processor. Blend until smooth and transfer to an ice cube tray. Freeze and store in zip-top bags, using cubes as needed.

3. Infusing Oils

- Infuse olive oil with fresh herbs for culinary uses. Simply submerge cleaned herbs in olive oil in a jar and let it sit in a cool, dark place for 1-2 weeks. Strain out the herbs and store the infused oil in a cool place.

4. Vinegar Infusions

- Similar to oil infusions, you can create flavorful herb-infused vinegar. Submerge fresh herbs in vinegar (such as apple cider or white wine vinegar) and let steep for a few weeks. Strain and store in a bottle.

Growing and harvesting your own medicinal herbs is a fulfilling way to connect with nature and enhance your health and wellness journey. By starting your herb garden, learning the proper techniques for harvesting, drying, and storing herbs, and mastering preservation methods, you can enjoy the benefits of fresh herbs year-round. Embrace this hands-on approach to herbal medicine, and cultivate a deeper appreciation for the healing power of plants in your daily life. With a little care and dedication, your garden can flourish, providing you with a continuous supply of the freshest, most potent herbal remedies right at your fingertips.

Chapter 20

Herbal Remedies for the Whole Family

Herbal remedies offer a natural approach to health and wellness that can benefit every member of the family, from children and pregnant women to seniors and pets. This chapter will explore safe herbal remedies tailored for specific age groups and life stages, provide pet-friendly herbal options, and share a soothing recipe for Calming Chamomile that can be enjoyed by both kids and pets.

Safe Remedies for Children, Pregnant Women, and Seniors

1. Herbal Remedies for Children

When using herbs for children, it's essential to choose gentle, safe options and consider appropriate dosages based on age. Here are some child-friendly herbs and their uses:

- **Chamomile**: Known for its calming properties, chamomile can help with sleep and soothe digestive issues.

- **Ginger**: A safe remedy for mild nausea and digestive discomfort, ginger can be given in tea or syrup form.

- **Peppermint**: This herb can alleviate tummy aches and headaches. Peppermint tea is a refreshing option for older children.

- **Echinacea**: Often used to boost the immune system, echinacea can help children recover from colds.

Dosage Guidelines:

- For children under 2 years: Use herbal remedies only under the guidance of a qualified healthcare provider.

- For children aged 2-12 years: Generally, a dosage of 1/4 to 1/2 of the adult dose is appropriate, but always consult with a healthcare provider for specific recommendations.

2. Herbal Remedies for Pregnant Women

Pregnancy is a time when caution is vital. Many herbs are safe during pregnancy, but others should be avoided. Here are some safe options:

- **Ginger**: Often used to alleviate morning sickness.

- **Peppermint**: Can help with nausea and digestive discomfort.

- **Raspberry Leaf**: Traditionally used to tone the uterus and support labor.

- **Lavender**: Known for its calming effects and can be used in aromatherapy to reduce anxiety.

Caution: Always consult with a healthcare provider before using any herbal remedies during pregnancy, as some herbs can have contraindications.

3. Herbal Remedies for Seniors

Seniors can benefit from herbal remedies, but considerations for medication interactions and health conditions are important. Here are some herbs that can be safe and effective:

- **Turmeric**: Known for its anti-inflammatory properties, it can help with joint pain and support overall health.

- **Ginkgo Biloba**: Often used to support cognitive function and improve circulation.

- **Valerian Root**: Can assist with sleep issues and anxiety.

- **Milk Thistle**: Supports liver health, which can be crucial for seniors.

Caution: Seniors should consult with a healthcare provider before starting new herbal remedies, especially if they are on multiple medications.

Pet-Friendly Herbal Remedies

Herbs can also be beneficial for our furry friends, but it's important to use them carefully. Here are some safe herbs for pets:

- **Chamomile**: Calming for both dogs and cats; it can help with anxiety and digestive issues.

- **Ginger**: Can be used to alleviate nausea and digestive discomfort in dogs.

- **Milk Thistle**: Supports liver health and is safe for both dogs and cats.

- **Peppermint**: May help freshen breath and soothe digestive upset in dogs (use in moderation).

Caution: Always consult with a veterinarian before administering herbal remedies to pets, as some herbs can be harmful to certain animals.

Recipe: Calming Chamomile for Kids and Pets

This soothing chamomile recipe is perfect for helping children and pets relax, especially before bedtime.

Ingredients:

- 1 tablespoon dried chamomile flowers (or 2 chamomile tea bags)

- 2 cups boiling water

- Honey (optional, for children over 1 year)

- A pinch of peppermint leaves (optional, for flavor)

Instructions:

1. **Prepare the Tea**:

    o Place the dried chamomile flowers or tea bags in a teapot or heatproof container.

o   Pour boiling water over the chamomile and let it steep for about 10 minutes.

2. **Strain the Tea**:

   o   If using loose flowers, strain the tea into cups. If using tea bags, simply remove them.

3. **Sweeten (Optional)**:

   o   For children over 1 year, add honey to taste. Avoid honey for children under 1 year due to the risk of botulism.

4. **Serve**:

   o   Allow the tea to cool to a safe temperature before serving to children or pets.

   o   For pets, serve the chamomile tea in a small bowl as a calming drink.

5. **Storage**:

   o   Store any leftover tea in the refrigerator for up to 48 hours. Reheat gently before serving.

Herbal remedies can be a safe and effective way to promote health and wellness for the entire family, including children, pregnant women, seniors, and even pets. By understanding which herbs are suitable for each group and using them responsibly, you can create a natural health toolkit that supports everyone's well-being. The Calming Chamomile recipe is just one example of how you can incorporate herbal remedies into daily life, fostering a sense of peace and relaxation for both your loved ones and furry friends. Embrace the power of herbal medicine and explore the many ways it can enrich your family's health and happiness.

Chapter 21

500 Natural Remedies for Every Ailment

1. Chamomile Tea

- **Uses:** Anxiety, insomnia, digestive issues.

- **Preparation:** Steep 1-2 teaspoons of dried chamomile flowers in hot water for 10 minutes. Strain and drink.

- **Benefits:** Calming effects, aids sleep, helps digestion.

- **Safety:** Generally safe, but may cause allergic reactions in those sensitive to ragweed.

2. Ginger Tea

- **Uses:** Nausea, digestion, inflammation.

- **Preparation:** Slice fresh ginger root and steep in boiling water for 10 minutes.

- **Benefits:** Eases nausea, promotes digestion, anti-inflammatory properties.

- **Safety:** High doses may cause heartburn; consult a doctor if pregnant.

3. Peppermint Oil

- **Uses:** Headaches, digestive issues, muscle pain.

- **Preparation:** Dilute peppermint oil with a carrier oil for topical use or inhale directly.

- **Benefits:** Relieves headaches, aids digestion, has a cooling effect on sore muscles.

- **Safety:** Avoid contact with eyes; may cause allergic reactions.

4. Turmeric

- **Uses:** Inflammation, joint pain, digestive issues.

- **Preparation:** Add powdered turmeric to meals or make a paste with water for topical use.

- **Benefits:** Strong anti-inflammatory and antioxidant properties.

- **Safety:** High doses may cause stomach upset; consult a doctor if on blood thinners.

5. Honey and Lemon

- **Uses:** Cough, sore throat, immune support.

- **Preparation:** Mix 1 tablespoon of honey and juice of half a lemon in warm water.

- **Benefits:** Soothes throat, boosts immune function.

- **Safety:** Do not give honey to children under 1 year.

6. Lavender Oil

- **Uses:** Anxiety, insomnia, skin irritation.

- **Preparation:** Use in a diffuser, dilute for topical use, or add to bathwater.

- **Benefits:** Promotes relaxation, improves sleep quality, soothing for the skin.

- **Safety:** Generally safe, but may cause skin irritation in some individuals.

7. Echinacea

- **Uses:** Immune support, cold prevention.

- **Preparation:** Use as a tincture, tea, or capsules.

- **Benefits:** Supports immune function, may reduce the duration of colds.

- **Safety:** May cause allergic reactions; avoid long-term use.

8. Aloe Vera

- **Uses:** Skin burns, hydration, digestive issues.

- **Preparation:** Apply fresh gel directly to the skin or consume in juice form.

- **Benefits:** Heals wounds, soothes burns, aids digestion.

- **Safety:** Overconsumption may lead to diarrhea.

9. Apple Cider Vinegar

- **Uses:** Digestive issues, weight loss, skin health.

- **Preparation:** Mix 1-2 tablespoons in a glass of water.

- **Benefits:** Supports digestion, balances pH, may aid weight loss.

- **Safety:** Can erode tooth enamel; always dilute.

10. Oatmeal Baths

- **Uses:** Skin irritation, eczema, dry skin.

- **Preparation:** Grind oats into a fine powder and add to bathwater.

- **Benefits:** Soothes itchy skin, hydrates.

- **Safety:** Generally safe; ensure oats are finely ground to avoid clogging drains.

11. Cinnamon

- **Uses:** Blood sugar control, digestive health.

- **Preparation:** Add to foods or drinks; cinnamon tea can be made by steeping sticks in water.

- **Benefits:** May help lower blood sugar levels, antibacterial properties.

- **Safety:** Cassia cinnamon can contain coumarin; use Ceylon cinnamon for safety.

12. Garlic

- **Uses:** Immune support, heart health.

- **Preparation:** Consume raw or add to meals; garlic oil can also be made.

- **Benefits:** Antimicrobial, heart-healthy properties.

- **Safety:** May cause digestive upset; can interact with blood thinners.

13. Thyme Tea

- **Uses:** Cough, respiratory issues.

- **Preparation:** Steep fresh or dried thyme in hot water.

- **Benefits:** Antiseptic, helps relieve coughs and bronchitis symptoms.

- **Safety:** Generally safe; large amounts may cause stomach upset.

14. Fennel Seeds

- **Uses:** Digestive health, bloating, gas.

- **Preparation:** Chew seeds directly or brew into a tea.

- **Benefits:** Relieves gas, aids digestion.

- **Safety:** Generally safe; excessive consumption may lead to hormonal effects.

15. Green Tea

- **Uses:** Antioxidant, metabolism boost.

- **Preparation:** Steep green tea leaves or bags in hot water.

- **Benefits:** High in antioxidants, may aid weight loss.

- **Safety:** High caffeine content; may cause insomnia or upset stomach.

16. Lemon Balm

- **Uses:** Anxiety, sleep issues, digestive problems.

- **Preparation:** Brew tea from fresh or dried leaves.

- **Benefits:** Calming effects, aids digestion.

- **Safety:** Generally safe; may cause drowsiness.

17. Bone Broth

- **Uses:** Gut health, joint pain.

- **Preparation:** Simmer bones with water and vinegar for 24 hours.

- **Benefits:** Rich in collagen and minerals, supports gut health.

* **Safety:** Ensure bones are sourced from healthy animals.

18. Cloves

* **Uses:** Toothache, digestive issues.

* **Preparation:** Use whole or ground in cooking, or make a clove tea.

* **Benefits:** Antiseptic properties, aids digestion.

* **Safety:** High doses may cause liver damage.

19. Basil

* **Uses:** Digestive aid, stress relief.

* **Preparation:** Use fresh or dried in cooking, or brew tea.

* **Benefits:** Antioxidant, may help reduce stress.

* **Safety:** Generally safe; large amounts may affect blood sugar levels.

20. Milk Thistle

* **Uses:** Liver health, detoxification.

* **Preparation:** Take as a supplement or brew tea from seeds.

* **Benefits:** Supports liver function, antioxidant effects.

* **Safety:** May cause gastrointestinal upset; consult a doctor if on medication.

21. Dandelion

* **Uses:** Liver health, digestive issues.

* **Preparation:** Use leaves in salads, brew roots for tea.

* **Benefits:** Supports liver and kidney health, aids digestion.

* **Safety:** May cause allergic reactions; consult a doctor if on diuretics.

22. St. John's Wort

- **Uses:** Mild depression, anxiety.

- **Preparation:** Take as a tea or supplement.

- **Benefits:** May help improve mood and reduce anxiety.

- **Safety:** Can interact with many medications; consult a healthcare provider.

23. Slippery Elm

- **Uses:** Digestive issues, sore throat.

- **Preparation:** Mix powder with water to form a paste or tea.

- **Benefits:** Soothes mucous membranes, aids digestion.

- **Safety:** Generally safe; may affect absorption of medications.

24. Nettle

- **Uses:** Allergies, inflammation.

- **Preparation:** Brew tea from fresh or dried leaves.

- **Benefits:** Anti-inflammatory, supports urinary health.

- **Safety:** Can cause skin irritation; avoid if allergic to plants in the Urticaceae family.

25. Black Cohosh

- **Uses:** Menopause symptoms.

- **Preparation:** Take as a supplement or brew tea.

- **Benefits:** May help alleviate hot flashes and mood swings.

- **Safety:** Consult a healthcare provider if pregnant or nursing.

26. Marshmallow Root

- **Uses:** Cough, sore throat, digestive issues.

- **Preparation:** Make tea or infuse in honey.

- **Benefits:** Soothes mucous membranes.

- **Safety:** Generally safe; may cause digestive upset in large amounts.

27. Cranberry Juice

- **Uses:** Urinary tract infections (UTIs).
- **Preparation:** Drink pure cranberry juice without added sugars.
- **Benefits:** Prevents bacteria from adhering to urinary tract walls.
- **Safety:** Large amounts may cause stomach upset; choose unsweetened.

28. Rosemary

- **Uses:** Memory enhancement, digestive health.
- **Preparation:** Use fresh or dried in cooking, or brew tea.
- **Benefits:** Antioxidant properties, may improve concentration.
- **Safety:** Generally safe; high doses may cause seizures.

29. Vitamin D

- **Uses:** Immune support, mood regulation.
- **Preparation:** Supplementation or sunlight exposure.
- **Benefits:** Supports immune function, mood stability.
- **Safety:** Excessive intake can lead to toxicity; consult a doctor for appropriate dosage.

30. Probiotics

- **Uses:** Gut health, immune support.
- **Preparation:** Consume fermented foods like yogurt, kefir, or take supplements.
- **Benefits:** Supports healthy gut flora, aids digestion.
- **Safety:** Generally safe; may cause bloating initially.

31. Hawthorn Berry

- **Uses:** Heart health, anxiety.

- **Preparation:** Use as a tincture, tea, or supplement.

- **Benefits:** Supports cardiovascular function.

- **Safety:** Consult a healthcare provider if on heart medications.

32. Licorice Root

- **Uses:** Sore throat, digestive health.

- **Preparation:** Brew tea or use in lozenges.

- **Benefits:** Soothing for throat, may aid digestion.

- **Safety:** Long-term use can lead to high blood pressure; consult a doctor if on medications.

33. Beetroot

- **Uses:** Blood pressure, stamina.

- **Preparation:** Consume raw, juiced, or cooked.

- **Benefits:** Supports cardiovascular health, boosts stamina.

- **Safety:** May cause beeturia (pink urine); generally safe.

34. Chia Seeds

- **Uses:** Digestive health, weight management.

- **Preparation:** Soak in water or add to smoothies and baked goods.

- **Benefits:** High in fiber and omega-3 fatty acids, aids digestion.

- **Safety:** May cause digestive upset if consumed dry.

35. Coconut Oil

- **Uses:** Skin health, digestive issues.

- **Preparation:** Use in cooking or apply topically.

- **Benefits:** Antimicrobial properties, moisturizing for skin.

- **Safety:** High in saturated fat; use in moderation.

36. Ashwagandha

- **Uses:** Stress, anxiety, fatigue.

- **Preparation:** Take as a powder or supplement.

- **Benefits:** Adaptogen, helps the body manage stress.

- **Safety:** May cause digestive upset; consult a doctor if on thyroid medications.

37. Cardamom

- **Uses:** Digestive health, respiratory issues.

- **Preparation:** Use whole or ground in cooking or tea.

- **Benefits:** Aids digestion, has antioxidant properties.

- **Safety:** Generally safe; excessive consumption may cause stomach upset.

38. Clary Sage

- **Uses:** Hormonal balance, stress relief.

- **Preparation:** Use essential oil in a diffuser or diluted for topical use.

- **Benefits:** May help with menstrual discomfort and anxiety.

- **Safety:** May cause allergic reactions; avoid if pregnant.

39. Ginseng

- **Uses:** Energy boost, stress relief.

- **Preparation:** Brew tea or take as a supplement.

- **Benefits:** Enhances energy, may improve focus.

- **Safety:** Can interact with blood thinners; consult a healthcare provider.

40. Sage

- **Uses:** Digestive health, sore throat.

- **Preparation:** Brew tea or use in cooking.

- **Benefits:** Antimicrobial, may soothe sore throats.

- **Safety:** Large amounts may have toxic effects; consult a doctor if pregnant.

41. Orange Peel

- **Uses:** Digestive aid, immune support.

- **Preparation:** Use fresh peel in teas or cooking.

- **Benefits:** High in vitamin C, aids digestion.

- **Safety:** Wash thoroughly before use to remove pesticides.

42. Moringa

- **Uses:** Nutrient boost, inflammation.

- **Preparation:** Take as a powder in smoothies or capsules.

- **Benefits:** High in vitamins and minerals, anti-inflammatory properties.

- **Safety:** Consult a doctor if pregnant; may lower blood sugar.

43. Thyme Essential Oil

- **Uses:** Respiratory issues, infections.

- **Preparation:** Dilute for topical use or use in a diffuser.

- **Benefits:** Antimicrobial, supports respiratory health.

- **Safety:** May irritate skin if used undiluted; avoid during pregnancy.

44. Ginkgo Biloba

- **Uses:** Memory support, circulation.

- **Preparation:** Take as a supplement or brew tea.

- **Benefits:** Improves circulation, may enhance cognitive function.

- **Safety:** Can interact with blood thinners; consult a healthcare provider.

45. Celery Seed

- **Uses:** Blood pressure, inflammation.

- **Preparation:** Use as a spice or take as a supplement.

- **Benefits:** May help lower blood pressure.

- **Safety:** Can cause allergic reactions; consult a doctor if pregnant.

46. Pumpkin Seeds

- **Uses:** Prostate health, digestion.

- **Preparation:** Eat raw or roasted.

- **Benefits:** Rich in zinc, supports prostate health.

- **Safety:** Generally safe; high in calories.

47. Red Clover

- **Uses:** Menopausal symptoms, blood health.

- **Preparation:** Brew tea or take as a supplement.

- **Benefits:** May alleviate hot flashes and improve circulation.

- **Safety:** Can interact with blood thinners; consult a healthcare provider.

48. Spirulina

- **Uses:** Nutrient boost, energy.

- **Preparation:** Take as a powder or in tablet form.

- **Benefits:** High in protein and nutrients, supports energy.

- **Safety:** May cause digestive upset; ensure sourced from clean waters.

49. Fenugreek

- **Uses:** Digestive aid, lactation support.

- **Preparation:** Use seeds in cooking or take as a supplement.

- **Benefits:** May improve digestion and boost milk production.

- **Safety:** Large amounts may cause diarrhea; consult a doctor if pregnant.

50. Thyroid-Boosting Herbs (e.g., Kelp)

- **Uses:** Thyroid health, metabolism.

- **Preparation:** Use in cooking or take as a supplement.

- **Benefits:** Source of iodine, supports thyroid function.

- **Safety:** Excessive iodine can lead to thyroid problems; consult a healthcare provider.

51. Flaxseeds

- **Uses:** Digestive health, heart health.

- **Preparation:** Consume ground seeds in smoothies, oatmeal, or yogurt.

- **Benefits:** High in omega-3 fatty acids and fiber; aids digestion and heart health.

- **Safety:** May cause digestive upset if consumed in large amounts; drink plenty of water.

52. Red Raspberry Leaf Tea

- **Uses:** Menstrual cramps, pregnancy support.

- **Preparation:** Brew dried leaves in hot water for 10 minutes.

- **Benefits:** Eases menstrual discomfort; may help tone the uterus during pregnancy.

- **Safety:** Generally safe; consult a healthcare provider if pregnant.

53. Holy Basil (Tulsi)

- **Uses:** Stress relief, immune support.

- **Preparation:** Brew tea from fresh or dried leaves.

- **Benefits:** Adaptogen that helps the body manage stress; boosts immunity.

- **Safety:** Generally safe; may interact with blood thinners.

54. Passionflower

- **Uses:** Anxiety, insomnia.

- **Preparation:** Brew tea from dried flowers or take as a supplement.

- **Benefits:** Calming effects, promotes better sleep.

- **Safety:** May cause drowsiness; avoid operating machinery after use.

55. Thyme

- **Uses:** Cough, respiratory health.

- **Preparation:** Steep fresh or dried thyme in hot water to make tea.

- **Benefits:** Antiseptic and expectorant properties; helps relieve coughs.

- **Safety:** Generally safe; avoid large amounts if allergic to Lamiaceae family.

56. Catnip

- **Uses:** Anxiety, digestive issues.

- **Preparation:** Brew tea from dried leaves.

- **Benefits:** Calming effects; aids digestion.

- **Safety:** Generally safe; may cause drowsiness.

57. Cod Liver Oil

- **Uses:** Joint health, immune support.

- **Preparation:** Consume as a liquid or in capsule form.

- **Benefits:** Rich in omega-3 fatty acids and vitamins A and D.

- **Safety:** High doses may lead to vitamin A toxicity; consult a healthcare provider.

58. Mullein

- **Uses:** Respiratory health, cough.

- **Preparation:** Brew tea from dried leaves or flowers.

- **Benefits:** Soothing for coughs and respiratory issues.

- **Safety:** Generally safe; avoid if allergic to plants in the Scrophulariaceae family.

59. Licorice Root Tea

- **Uses:** Sore throat, digestive issues.

- **Preparation:** Steep dried licorice root in hot water.

- **Benefits:** Soothes throat; may aid digestion.

- **Safety:** Long-term use can cause high blood pressure; consult a doctor if on medications.

60. Barley Grass Juice

- **Uses:** Nutrient boost, detoxification.

- **Preparation:** Juice fresh barley grass or take as a powder.

- **Benefits:** Rich in vitamins, minerals, and antioxidants; supports detoxification.

- **Safety:** Generally safe; consult a healthcare provider if on anticoagulants.

61. Burdock Root

- **Uses:** Blood purification, skin health.

- **Preparation:** Brew tea from dried root or use in soups.

- **Benefits:** Aids liver function and improves skin health.

- **Safety:** Generally safe; large amounts may cause digestive upset.

62. Chervil

- **Uses:** Digestive aid, nutrient boost.

- **Preparation:** Use fresh in salads or as a seasoning.

- **Benefits:** Promotes digestion; rich in vitamins.

- **Safety:** Generally safe; may cause allergic reactions in some individuals.

63. Juniper Berries

- **Uses:** Digestive health, urinary tract health.

- **Preparation:** Use whole berries in cooking or brew as tea.

- **Benefits:** Aids digestion and may support urinary health.

- **Safety:** Not recommended for pregnant women; excessive consumption may irritate the kidneys.

64. Anise Seed

- **Uses:** Digestive issues, respiratory health.

- **Preparation:** Brew tea from seeds or use in cooking.

- **Benefits:** Relieves bloating and gas; soothes coughs.

- **Safety:** Generally safe; may cause allergic reactions in some individuals.

65. Neem

- **Uses:** Skin health, immune support.

- **Preparation:** Use neem oil or make tea from leaves.

- **Benefits:** Antimicrobial and anti-inflammatory properties; supports skin health.

- **Safety:** May cause skin irritation; avoid if allergic to the Meliaceae family.

66. Jojoba Oil

- **Uses:** Skin hydration, hair care.

- **Preparation:** Apply directly to skin or hair as needed.

- **Benefits:** Moisturizes without clogging pores; nourishes hair.

- **Safety:** Generally safe; may cause allergic reactions in some individuals.

67. Maca Root

- **Uses:** Energy boost, hormonal balance.

- **Preparation:** Take as a powder in smoothies or capsules.

- **Benefits:** Boosts energy, may improve mood and hormonal balance.

- **Safety:** Generally safe; consult a healthcare provider if pregnant or nursing.

68. Artichoke Leaf Extract

- **Uses:** Digestive health, cholesterol support.

- **Preparation:** Take as a supplement or extract.

- **Benefits:** Supports liver function and helps lower cholesterol levels.

- **Safety:** May cause digestive upset; consult a healthcare provider if on medications.

69. Rosemary Oil

- **Uses:** Memory enhancement, hair growth.

- **Preparation:** Dilute for topical use or use in a diffuser.

- **Benefits:** May improve memory and promote hair growth.

- **Safety:** May cause skin irritation; avoid if pregnant.

70. Schisandra Berry

- **Uses:** Stress relief, liver health.

- **Preparation:** Take as a supplement or brew tea.

- **Benefits:** Adaptogen; supports liver function and stress resilience.

- **Safety:** Generally safe; consult a healthcare provider if on blood pressure medications.

71. Yellow Dock Root

- **Uses:** Digestive health, skin issues.

- **Preparation:** Brew tea from dried root.

- **Benefits:** Aids digestion; may improve skin health.

- **Safety:** Generally safe; excessive use may cause digestive upset.

72. Cilantro

- **Uses:** Heavy metal detoxification, digestion.

- **Preparation:** Use fresh in salads, smoothies, or cooking.

- **Benefits:** May help remove heavy metals from the body.

- **Safety:** Generally safe; excessive amounts may cause digestive upset.

73. Seaweed (Kombu, Nori)

- **Uses:** Thyroid health, nutrient boost.

- **Preparation:** Use in soups or salads; available in dried sheets.

- **Benefits:** Rich in iodine, supports thyroid function.

- **Safety:** Excessive consumption may lead to iodine toxicity; consult a healthcare provider.

74. Valerian Root

- **Uses:** Insomnia, anxiety.

- **Preparation:** Brew tea or take as a supplement.

- **Benefits:** Calming effects; promotes better sleep.

- **Safety:** May cause drowsiness; avoid operating machinery after use.

75. Dulse

- **Uses:** Nutrient boost, thyroid health.

- **Preparation:** Use dried flakes in salads or soups.

- **Benefits:** Rich in minerals, including iodine; supports thyroid function.

- **Safety:** May cause digestive upset; excessive intake can lead to iodine toxicity.

76. Collagen Supplements

- **Uses:** Joint health, skin elasticity.

- **Preparation:** Consume as a powder in drinks or capsules.

- **Benefits:** Supports joint health and improves skin elasticity.

- **Safety:** Generally safe; consult a healthcare provider if allergic to shellfish.

77. Hops

- **Uses:** Anxiety, insomnia.

- **Preparation:** Brew tea or take as a supplement.

- **Benefits:** Calming effects; may improve sleep quality.

- **Safety:** May cause drowsiness; avoid operating machinery after use.

78. Fenugreek Tea

- **Uses:** Lactation support, digestive health.

- **Preparation:** Steep seeds in hot water.

- **Benefits:** May increase milk production and support digestion.

- **Safety:** Generally safe; large amounts may cause diarrhea.

79. Soursop

- **Uses:** Immune support, digestive health.

- **Preparation:** Consume fresh fruit or drink juice.

- **Benefits:** Rich in antioxidants; may help boost immunity.

- **Safety:** Consult a healthcare provider if pregnant or nursing.

80. Clary Sage Oil

- **Uses:** Hormonal balance, stress relief.
- **Preparation:** Use diluted for topical application or in a diffuser.
- **Benefits:** May alleviate menstrual discomfort and reduce anxiety.
- **Safety:** May cause skin irritation; avoid during pregnancy.

81. Burdock Leaf Tea

- **Uses:** Skin health, detoxification.
- **Preparation:** Brew dried leaves in hot water.
- **Benefits:** Supports skin health and liver function.
- **Safety:** Generally safe; avoid large amounts.

82. Black Seed Oil (Nigella sativa)

- **Uses:** Immune support, inflammation.
- **Preparation:** Take as a supplement or use in cooking.
- **Benefits:** Anti-inflammatory and antioxidant properties.
- **Safety:** Generally safe; may interact with certain medications.

83. Red Clover Tea

- **Uses:** Hormonal balance, skin health.
- **Preparation:** Brew dried flowers in hot water.
- **Benefits:** May alleviate menopausal symptoms; supports skin health.
- **Safety:** Can interact with blood thinners; consult a healthcare provider.

84. Ginger Tea

- **Uses:** Nausea, digestive health.
- **Preparation:** Steep fresh ginger slices in hot water.

- **Benefits:** Eases nausea and aids digestion.

- **Safety:** Generally safe; may cause heartburn in some individuals.

85. Lemon Balm

- **Uses:** Anxiety, digestive issues.

- **Preparation:** Brew tea from fresh or dried leaves.

- **Benefits:** Calming effects; supports digestion.

- **Safety:** Generally safe; may cause allergic reactions in some individuals.

86. Nettle

- **Uses:** Allergies, joint health.

- **Preparation:** Brew tea from dried leaves or use in soups.

- **Benefits:** May alleviate allergy symptoms; supports joint health.

- **Safety:** Generally safe; may cause skin irritation if handled fresh.

87. Kava Kava

- **Uses:** Anxiety, relaxation.

- **Preparation:** Brew tea from the root or take as a supplement.

- **Benefits:** Calming effects; promotes relaxation and stress relief.

- **Safety:** May cause liver damage with excessive use; consult a healthcare provider.

88. Astragalus

- **Uses:** Immune support, stress resilience.

- **Preparation:** Brew tea from dried root or take as a supplement.

- **Benefits:** Boosts immune function; supports stress resilience.

- **Safety:** Generally safe; consult a healthcare provider if on immunosuppressants.

89. Chamomile

- **Uses:** Sleep aid, digestive issues.

- **Preparation:** Brew tea from dried flowers.

- **Benefits:** Calming effects; aids digestion and promotes sleep.

- **Safety:** May cause allergic reactions; avoid if allergic to Asteraceae family.

90. Dandelion

- **Uses:** Digestive health, liver support.

- **Preparation:** Brew tea from leaves or roots.

- **Benefits:** Supports liver function; aids digestion.

- **Safety:** Generally safe; avoid if allergic to related plants.

91. Arjuna (Terminalia arjuna)

- **Uses:** Heart health, blood pressure.

- **Preparation:** Take as a supplement or brew tea.

- **Benefits:** Supports cardiovascular health; may help lower blood pressure.

- **Safety:** Generally safe; consult a healthcare provider if on blood pressure medications.

92. Grape Seed Extract

- **Uses:** Antioxidant support, heart health.

- **Preparation:** Take as a supplement.

- **Benefits:** Rich in antioxidants; supports cardiovascular health.

- **Safety:** Generally safe; may interact with certain medications.

93. Maca Root Powder

- **Uses:** Hormonal balance, energy.

- **Preparation:** Add to smoothies, oatmeal, or baked goods.

- **Benefits:** May enhance energy and balance hormones.

- **Safety:** Generally safe; consult a healthcare provider if pregnant.

94. Caraway Seeds

- **Uses:** Digestive issues, respiratory health.

- **Preparation:** Use in cooking or brew tea.

- **Benefits:** Aids digestion; may relieve respiratory issues.

- **Safety:** Generally safe; excessive amounts may cause digestive upset.

95. Cucumber

- **Uses:** Hydration, skin health.

- **Preparation:** Eat raw in salads or juice.

- **Benefits:** Hydrating and rich in antioxidants; supports skin health.

- **Safety:** Generally safe; wash thoroughly to remove pesticides.

96. Licorice Root Capsules

- **Uses:** Digestive health, respiratory issues.

- **Preparation:** Take as directed on the label.

- **Benefits:** Soothes digestive tract; may relieve coughs.

- **Safety:** Long-term use can lead to high blood pressure; consult a doctor.

97. Macadamia Nut Oil

- **Uses:** Skin hydration, hair care.

- **Preparation:** Apply topically or use in cooking.

- **Benefits:** Rich in fatty acids; moisturizes skin and hair.

- **Safety:** Generally safe; high in calories.

98. Oregano Oil

- **Uses:** Antimicrobial, respiratory health.

- **Preparation:** Use diluted for topical application or in a diffuser.

- **Benefits:** Antibacterial and antiviral properties; supports respiratory health.

- **Safety:** May irritate skin if used undiluted; consult a healthcare provider.

99. Elderflower

- **Uses:** Immune support, respiratory health.

- **Preparation:** Brew tea from dried flowers.

- **Benefits:** May help reduce cold symptoms; boosts immunity.

- **Safety:** Generally safe; avoid if allergic to related plants.

100. Yarrow

- **Uses:** Wound healing, digestive health.

- **Preparation:** Brew tea or apply crushed leaves to wounds.

- **Benefits:** Promotes healing of wounds; supports digestion.

- **Safety:** May cause allergic reactions; avoid if pregnant.

101. Aloe Vera

- **Uses:** Skin burns, digestive health.

- **Preparation:** Apply gel directly from the leaf or consume juice.

- **Benefits:** Soothes burns and promotes skin healing; may aid digestion.

- **Safety:** Generally safe; may cause diarrhea if taken in large amounts.

102. Ashwagandha

- **Uses:** Stress relief, energy boost.

- **Preparation:** Take as a powder, capsule, or tincture.

- **Benefits:** Adaptogen that reduces stress and enhances energy.

- **Safety:** Generally safe; consult a healthcare provider if pregnant.

103. Black Cohosh

- **Uses:** Menopause symptoms, menstrual cramps.

- **Preparation:** Take as a supplement or brew tea.

- **Benefits:** May alleviate hot flashes and menstrual discomfort.

- **Safety:** Consult a healthcare provider if on hormone therapy; may cause liver issues in rare cases.

104. Moringa

- **Uses:** Nutritional support, energy booster.

- **Preparation:** Consume powder in smoothies or capsules.

- **Benefits:** Rich in vitamins and minerals; boosts energy levels.

- **Safety:** Generally safe; large amounts may cause digestive upset.

105. Cacao Nibs

- **Uses:** Mood enhancement, heart health.

- **Preparation:** Add to smoothies, oatmeal, or eat raw.

- **Benefits:** Rich in antioxidants; may improve mood and heart health.

- **Safety:** Generally safe; excessive consumption may lead to caffeine-related side effects.

106. Oregano

- **Uses:** Antimicrobial, respiratory health.

- **Preparation:** Use fresh or dried in cooking or make tea.

- **Benefits:** Antibacterial and antifungal properties; may relieve respiratory issues.

- **Safety:** Generally safe; large amounts may cause gastrointestinal upset.

107. Fenugreek Seeds

- **Uses:** Lactation support, blood sugar regulation.

- **Preparation:** Soak seeds overnight, grind, and add to food or brew tea.

- **Benefits:** May help increase milk production and regulate blood sugar levels.

- **Safety:** Generally safe; consult a healthcare provider if pregnant.

108. Bilberry

- **Uses:** Eye health, circulation.

- **Preparation:** Take as a supplement or consume fresh berries.

- **Benefits:** Rich in antioxidants; supports eye health and improves circulation.

- **Safety:** Generally safe; large amounts may cause digestive upset.

109. Ginseng

- **Uses:** Energy, cognitive function.

- **Preparation:** Brew tea from root or take as a supplement.

- **Benefits:** Boosts energy and may enhance cognitive function.

- **Safety:** Generally safe; avoid large doses; may interact with blood thinners.

110. Ginkgo Biloba

- **Uses:** Memory enhancement, circulation.

- **Preparation:** Take as a supplement or brew tea.

- **Benefits:** May improve memory and enhance blood flow.

- **Safety:** Generally safe; may cause digestive upset; consult a healthcare provider if on anticoagulants.

111. Cinnamon

- **Uses:** Blood sugar regulation, digestive health.

- **Preparation:** Use ground cinnamon in cooking or brew tea.

- **Benefits:** May help lower blood sugar levels and improve digestion.

- **Safety:** Generally safe; excessive amounts may cause liver issues.

112. Nutmeg

- **Uses:** Digestive health, sleep aid.

- **Preparation:** Use ground in cooking or brew tea.

- **Benefits:** Aids digestion and promotes relaxation.

- **Safety:** Generally safe in culinary amounts; excessive use may cause hallucinations or toxicity.

113. Coconut Oil

- **Uses:** Skin hydration, hair care.

- **Preparation:** Apply topically or use in cooking.

- **Benefits:** Moisturizes skin and hair; contains antibacterial properties.

- **Safety:** Generally safe; high in saturated fats; use in moderation.

114. Cabbage

- **Uses:** Digestive health, skin health.

- **Preparation:** Eat raw in salads or juice.

- **Benefits:** Rich in vitamins and fiber; promotes gut health.

- **Safety:** Generally safe; excessive consumption may cause gas.

115. Butternut Squash

- **Uses:** Digestive health, skin health.

- **Preparation:** Roast, steam, or puree.

- **Benefits:** High in fiber and antioxidants; supports skin health and digestion.

- **Safety:** Generally safe; consult a healthcare provider if allergic.

116. Marshmallow Root

- **Uses:** Sore throat, digestive health.

- **Preparation:** Brew tea from dried root.

- **Benefits:** Soothes throat and may help with digestive issues.

- **Safety:** Generally safe; large amounts may cause digestive upset.

117. Prickly Pear

- **Uses:** Blood sugar regulation, digestive health.

- **Preparation:** Eat raw or juice the pads and fruit.

- **Benefits:** High in fiber; may help regulate blood sugar levels.

- **Safety:** Generally safe; may cause digestive upset in some individuals.

118. Lemongrass

- **Uses:** Digestive health, stress relief.

- **Preparation:** Brew tea from fresh or dried leaves.

- **Benefits:** Aids digestion and has calming effects.

- **Safety:** Generally safe; excessive amounts may cause digestive upset.

119. Thyme Oil

- **Uses:** Antimicrobial, respiratory health.

- **Preparation:** Dilute for topical use or diffuse.

- **Benefits:** Antibacterial properties; supports respiratory function.

- **Safety:** May cause skin irritation if used undiluted; avoid during pregnancy.

120. Chia Seeds

- **Uses:** Digestive health, energy boost.

- **Preparation:** Soak in water or add to smoothies and oatmeal.

- **Benefits:** High in omega-3s and fiber; promotes fullness and digestive health.

- **Safety:** Generally safe; increase intake gradually to avoid digestive upset.

121. Dandelion Root Coffee

- **Uses:** Liver health, digestive support.

- **Preparation:** Roast dried roots and brew as coffee.

- **Benefits:** Supports liver function and aids digestion.

- **Safety:** Generally safe; excessive consumption may cause digestive upset.

122. Green Tea

- **Uses:** Antioxidant support, metabolism boost.

- **Preparation:** Brew tea from leaves or consume as extract.

- **Benefits:** Rich in antioxidants; may aid weight loss and boost metabolism.

- **Safety:** Generally safe; excessive caffeine may lead to insomnia or jitters.

123. Saffron

- **Uses:** Mood enhancement, menstrual support.

- **Preparation:** Steep threads in warm water or milk.

- **Benefits:** May improve mood and alleviate menstrual symptoms.

- **Safety:** Generally safe; excessive amounts can be toxic.

124. Wheatgrass

- **Uses:** Nutrient boost, detoxification.

- **Preparation:** Juice fresh wheatgrass or consume as powder.

- **Benefits:** Rich in vitamins and minerals; supports detoxification.

- **Safety:** Generally safe; may cause nausea in some individuals.

125. Red Clover

- **Uses:** Hormonal balance, skin health.

- **Preparation:** Brew tea from dried flowers.

- **Benefits:** May alleviate menopausal symptoms and improve skin health.

- **Safety:** Generally safe; may interact with blood thinners.

126. Black Garlic

- **Uses:** Immune support, cardiovascular health.

- **Preparation:** Consume raw or add to dishes.

- **Benefits:** Rich in antioxidants; may support heart health.

- **Safety:** Generally safe; excessive consumption may cause digestive upset.

127. Kelp

- **Uses:** Thyroid health, nutrient boost.

- **Preparation:** Use dried flakes in cooking or take as a supplement.

- **Benefits:** High in iodine; supports thyroid function.

- **Safety:** Excessive intake can lead to iodine toxicity; consult a healthcare provider.

128. Quinoa

- **Uses:** Nutritional support, digestive health.

- **Preparation:** Cook as a grain in water.

- **Benefits:** High in protein and fiber; promotes digestive health.

- **Safety:** Generally safe; wash thoroughly to remove saponins.

129. Hops Extract

- **Uses:** Anxiety, sleep aid.

- **Preparation:** Take as a supplement or brew tea.

- **Benefits:** Promotes relaxation and better sleep quality.

- **Safety:** May cause drowsiness; avoid operating machinery after use.

130. Rosehip

- **Uses:** Skin health, joint health.

- **Preparation:** Brew tea or consume as a supplement.

- **Benefits:** High in vitamin C; supports skin and joint health.

- **Safety:** Generally safe; excessive amounts may cause digestive upset.

131. Ginger Oil

- **Uses:** Nausea, inflammation.

- **Preparation:** Dilute for topical use or use in aromatherapy.

- **Benefits:** May relieve nausea and reduce inflammation.

- **Safety:** May cause skin irritation if used undiluted; consult a healthcare provider if pregnant.

132. Arugula

- **Uses:** Digestive health, nutrient boost.

- **Preparation:** Use fresh in salads or smoothies.

- **Benefits:** High in vitamins and minerals; promotes digestive health.

- **Safety:** Generally safe; excessive consumption may cause digestive upset.

133. Soursop Leaves

- **Uses:** Immune support, anti-inflammatory.

- **Preparation:** Brew tea from dried leaves.

- **Benefits:** May help reduce inflammation and boost immunity.

- **Safety:** Generally safe; excessive consumption may have adverse effects.

134. Star Anise

- **Uses:** Digestive health, respiratory health.

- **Preparation:** Use in cooking or brew tea.

- **Benefits:** Aids digestion and may relieve coughs.

- **Safety:** Generally safe; avoid large amounts as they can be toxic.

135. Flaxseed

- **Uses:** Digestive health, hormonal balance.

- **Preparation:** Ground and added to foods or consumed as oil.

- **Benefits:** High in omega-3s; promotes digestive health and hormonal balance.

- **Safety:** Generally safe; excessive amounts may cause digestive upset.

136. Cilantro

- **Uses:** Detoxification, digestive health.

- **Preparation:** Use fresh in salads or cooking.

- **Benefits:** May help remove heavy metals from the body; supports digestion.

- **Safety:** Generally safe; avoid if allergic to related plants.

137. Turmeric Curcumin

- **Uses:** Inflammation, joint health.

- **Preparation:** Take as a supplement or add to cooking.

- **Benefits:** Strong anti-inflammatory properties; supports joint health.

- **Safety:** Generally safe; may cause digestive upset in large doses.

138. Catnip

- **Uses:** Anxiety, sleep aid.

- **Preparation:** Brew tea from dried leaves.

- **Benefits:** Calming effects; may promote better sleep.

- **Safety:** Generally safe; excessive consumption may cause mild gastrointestinal issues.

139. Sweet Basil

- **Uses:** Digestive health, stress relief.

- **Preparation:** Use fresh in cooking or brew tea.

- **Benefits:** Aids digestion and has calming properties.

- **Safety:** Generally safe; excessive amounts may cause digestive upset.

140. Pineapple

- **Uses:** Digestive health, inflammation.

- **Preparation:** Eat raw or juice.

- **Benefits:** Contains bromelain, which aids digestion and reduces inflammation.

- **Safety:** Generally safe; may cause allergic reactions in some individuals.

141. Celery Seed

- **Uses:** Blood pressure, anti-inflammatory.

- **Preparation:** Use as a spice or take as a supplement.

- **Benefits:** May help lower blood pressure and reduce inflammation.

- **Safety:** Generally safe; large amounts may cause digestive upset.

142. Rosemary

- **Uses:** Cognitive function, digestion.

- **Preparation:** Use fresh or dried in cooking or brew tea.

- **Benefits:** May enhance memory and improve digestion.

- **Safety:** Generally safe; excessive amounts may cause digestive upset.

143. Scullcap

- **Uses:** Anxiety, sleep aid.

- **Preparation:** Brew tea from dried leaves.

- **Benefits:** Calming effects; promotes relaxation and sleep.

- **Safety:** Generally safe; may cause drowsiness; avoid operating machinery after use.

144. Fennel Seeds

- **Uses:** Digestive issues, respiratory health.

- **Preparation:** Chew seeds or brew tea.

- **Benefits:** Aids digestion and may relieve coughs.

- **Safety:** Generally safe; excessive consumption may cause digestive upset.

145. Sea Buckthorn Oil

- **Uses:** Skin health, immune support.

- **Preparation:** Apply topically or take as a supplement.

- **Benefits:** Rich in vitamins and antioxidants; supports skin health and immunity.

- **Safety:** Generally safe; consult a healthcare provider for dosage.

146. Bitter Melon

- **Uses:** Blood sugar regulation, digestive health.

- **Preparation:** Consume raw or in cooking.

- **Benefits:** May help lower blood sugar levels and support digestion.

- **Safety:** Consult a healthcare provider if diabetic; may interact with blood sugar medications.

147. Chamomile Oil

- **Uses:** Anxiety, skin irritations.

- **Preparation:** Dilute for topical use or use in aromatherapy.

- **Benefits:** Soothes skin and promotes relaxation.

- **Safety:** May cause allergic reactions; avoid if allergic to Asteraceae family.

148. Goat's Rue

- **Uses:** Lactation support, blood sugar regulation.

- **Preparation:** Brew tea from dried leaves.

- **Benefits:** May help increase milk production and regulate blood sugar levels.

- **Safety:** Consult a healthcare provider if pregnant.

149. Blueberry

- **Uses:** Antioxidant support, heart health.

- **Preparation:** Eat raw, add to smoothies or baked goods.

- **Benefits:** High in antioxidants; supports heart and brain health.

- **Safety:** Generally safe; wash thoroughly to remove pesticides.

150. Cardamom

- **Uses:** Digestive health, respiratory health.

- **Preparation:** Use whole pods in cooking or brew tea.

- **Benefits:** Aids digestion and may relieve coughs.

- **Safety:** Generally safe; excessive amounts may cause digestive upset.

151. Nettle Leaf

- **Uses:** Allergy relief, anti-inflammatory.

- **Preparation:** Brew tea from dried leaves or consume capsules.

- **Benefits:** May reduce symptoms of hay fever and inflammation.

- **Safety:** Generally safe; may cause stomach upset in some individuals.

152. Cloves

- **Uses:** Toothache relief, digestive aid.

- **Preparation:** Chew whole cloves or use clove oil.

- **Benefits:** Contains eugenol, which may alleviate tooth pain; aids digestion.

- **Safety:** Generally safe; excessive amounts can cause gastrointestinal irritation.

153. Licorice Root

- **Uses:** Sore throat, adrenal support.

- **Preparation:** Brew tea or take as a supplement.

- **Benefits:** Soothes throat and may help with adrenal fatigue.

- **Safety:** Prolonged use may cause high blood pressure; consult a healthcare provider.

154. Sage

- **Uses:** Digestive health, sore throat relief.

- **Preparation:** Brew tea from fresh or dried leaves.

- **Benefits:** Aids digestion and has antimicrobial properties.

- **Safety:** Generally safe; avoid large amounts during pregnancy.

155. Passionflower

- **Uses:** Anxiety, sleep disorders.

- **Preparation:** Brew tea from dried flowers or take as a supplement.

- **Benefits:** May help reduce anxiety and promote better sleep.

- **Safety:** Generally safe; may cause drowsiness; avoid operating machinery after use.

156. Neem

- **Uses:** Skin conditions, dental health.

- **Preparation:** Use neem oil or extract topically; consume capsules.

- **Benefits:** Antimicrobial properties; may help with acne and oral health.

- **Safety:** Generally safe; excessive oral consumption may cause toxicity.

157. Echinacea

- **Uses:** Immune support, cold prevention.

- **Preparation:** Brew tea or take as a supplement.

- **Benefits:** May boost the immune system and reduce cold duration.

- **Safety:** Generally safe; avoid in autoimmune disorders.

158. Rhodiola Rosea

- **Uses:** Stress relief, fatigue.

- **Preparation:** Take as a supplement or tincture.

- **Benefits:** Adaptogen that may help reduce fatigue and improve mood.

- **Safety:** Generally safe; may cause dizziness or dry mouth.

159. Holy Basil (Tulsi)

- **Uses:** Stress relief, immune support.

- **Preparation:** Brew tea from fresh or dried leaves.

- **Benefits:** Adaptogen that may help balance stress and support immunity.

- **Safety:** Generally safe; consult a healthcare provider if pregnant.

160. Yellow Dock Root

- **Uses:** Digestive health, liver support.

- **Preparation:** Brew tea or take as a supplement.

- **Benefits:** May support liver function and aid digestion.

- **Safety:** Generally safe; excessive amounts may cause digestive upset.

161. Chaga Mushroom

- **Uses:** Immune support, antioxidant boost.

- **Preparation:** Brew tea or take as a supplement.

- **Benefits:** High in antioxidants; may boost immunity.

- **Safety:** Generally safe; may interact with anticoagulants.

162. Willow Bark

- **Uses:** Pain relief, inflammation.

- **Preparation:** Brew tea or take as a supplement.

- **Benefits:** Contains salicin, which may relieve pain and reduce inflammation.

- **Safety:** Generally safe; may cause stomach upset.

163. Sea Moss

- **Uses:** Nutritional support, thyroid health.

- **Preparation:** Consume raw, dried, or in smoothies.

- **Benefits:** Rich in vitamins and minerals; supports thyroid function.

- **Safety:** Generally safe; ensure proper sourcing to avoid contaminants.

164. Spirulina

- **Uses:** Nutritional boost, immune support.

- **Preparation:** Consume as powder in smoothies or as tablets.

- **Benefits:** High in protein and nutrients; may boost immunity.

- **Safety:** Generally safe; may cause digestive upset in some individuals.

165. Maca Root

- **Uses:** Energy, hormonal balance.

- **Preparation:** Consume as powder in smoothies or capsules.

- **Benefits:** May enhance energy levels and improve hormonal balance.

- **Safety:** Generally safe; may cause digestive upset in some individuals.

166. Dandelion Greens

- **Uses:** Detoxification, digestive health.

- **Preparation:** Use fresh in salads or smoothies.

- **Benefits:** High in vitamins; supports liver health and digestion.

- **Safety:** Generally safe; avoid if allergic to related plants.

167. Cardamom

- **Uses:** Digestive health, respiratory health.

- **Preparation:** Use ground or whole pods in cooking or brew tea.

- **Benefits:** Aids digestion and may relieve coughs.

- **Safety:** Generally safe; excessive amounts may cause digestive upset.

168. Horse Chestnut

- **Uses:** Circulation, varicose veins.

- **Preparation:** Take as a supplement or apply topical extract.

- **Benefits:** May improve circulation and reduce swelling.

- **Safety:** Generally safe; may cause stomach upset; consult a healthcare provider.

169. Tumeric (Curcumin)

- **Uses:** Inflammation, joint health.

- **Preparation:** Use fresh, powdered in cooking, or as a supplement.

- **Benefits:** Powerful anti-inflammatory properties; supports joint health.

- **Safety:** Generally safe; large doses may cause digestive upset.

170. Bitter Orange

- **Uses:** Digestive health, appetite suppressant.

- **Preparation:** Use in tea or as a supplement.

- **Benefits:** May aid digestion and help with weight management.

- **Safety:** May increase heart rate; consult a healthcare provider if on medications.

171. Burdock Root

- **Uses:** Skin health, detoxification.

- **Preparation:** Brew tea or consume cooked.

- **Benefits:** May help with skin issues and detoxify the body.

- **Safety:** Generally safe; may cause digestive upset in some individuals.

172. Rosewater

- **Uses:** Skin hydration, mood enhancement.

- **Preparation:** Use as a toner or in cooking.

- **Benefits:** Hydrates skin and may improve mood with aroma.

- **Safety:** Generally safe; ensure no allergies to roses.

173. Yellow Dock Root

- **Uses:** Digestive health, liver support.

- **Preparation:** Brew tea or take as a supplement.

- **Benefits:** May support liver function and promote digestion.

- **Safety:** Generally safe; large amounts may cause stomach upset.

174. Coriander

- **Uses:** Digestive aid, detoxification.

- **Preparation:** Use fresh leaves or seeds in cooking.

- **Benefits:** May help with digestion and heavy metal detoxification.

- **Safety:** Generally safe; avoid large amounts if allergic.

175. Hawthorn Berries

- **Uses:** Heart health, circulation.

- **Preparation:** Brew tea or take as a supplement.

- **Benefits:** May improve heart function and circulation.

- **Safety:** Generally safe; consult a healthcare provider if on heart medications.

176. Coconut Water

- **Uses:** Hydration, electrolyte balance.

- **Preparation:** Drink raw from coconuts or in cartons.

- **Benefits:** Natural electrolyte source; hydrates the body.

- **Safety:** Generally safe; high in potassium; consult a healthcare provider if on potassium-restricted diets.

177. Lavender

- **Uses:** Anxiety, sleep aid.

- **Preparation:** Use essential oil for aromatherapy or brew tea.

- **Benefits:** Calming properties; promotes relaxation and better sleep.

- **Safety:** Generally safe; may cause skin irritation in some.

178. Beets

- **Uses:** Blood pressure, liver health.

- **Preparation:** Cooked, juiced, or consumed raw.

- **Benefits:** May help lower blood pressure and support liver health.

- **Safety:** Generally safe; high oxalate content; consult a healthcare provider if prone to kidney stones.

179. Kava Kava

- **Uses:** Anxiety, stress relief.

- **Preparation:** Brew tea or take as a supplement.

- **Benefits:** Calming effects; may reduce anxiety levels.

- **Safety:** Potential liver toxicity; consult a healthcare provider before use.

180. Cucumber

- **Uses:** Hydration, skin health.

- **Preparation:** Eat raw in salads or as juice.

- **Benefits:** High in water content; hydrates skin and body.

- **Safety:** Generally safe; wash thoroughly to avoid pesticides.

181. Persimmon

- **Uses:** Digestive health, antioxidant support.

- **Preparation:** Eat raw or dried.

- **Benefits:** High in fiber and antioxidants; promotes digestive health.

- **Safety:** Generally safe; excessive consumption may cause constipation.

182. Black Seed Oil

- **Uses:** Immune support, skin health.

- **Preparation:** Take as a supplement or apply topically.

- **Benefits:** Contains thymoquinone, which may enhance immunity and improve skin health.

- **Safety:** Generally safe; consult a healthcare provider if pregnant.

183. Ginger Ale (Natural)

- **Uses:** Nausea, digestive aid.

- **Preparation:** Make with fresh ginger, lemon, and carbonated water.

- **Benefits:** Soothes nausea and aids digestion.

- **Safety:** Generally safe; excessive sugar can negate health benefits.

184. Sweet Potatoes

- **Uses:** Nutritional support, digestive health.

- **Preparation:** Roast, steam, or mash.

- **Benefits:** High in vitamins and fiber; supports digestive health.

- **Safety:** Generally safe; consult a healthcare provider for personalized dietary advice.

185. Cardamom

- **Uses:** Digestive health, respiratory health.

- **Preparation:** Use as a spice or brew tea.

- **Benefits:** May aid digestion and relieve coughs.

- **Safety:** Generally safe; excessive consumption may cause digestive upset.

186. Apricot Kernels

- **Uses:** Antioxidant support, cancer prevention (controversial).

- **Preparation:** Consume raw or in oil form.

- **Benefits:** High in vitamin B17; promotes overall health.

- **Safety:** May contain cyanide; consult a healthcare provider before use.

187. Mulberries

- **Uses:** Nutritional support, blood sugar regulation.

- **Preparation:** Eat raw, dried, or in smoothies.

- **Benefits:** High in vitamins; may help regulate blood sugar.

- **Safety:** Generally safe; wash thoroughly to remove pesticides.

188. Gooseberry (Amla)

- **Uses:** Antioxidant support, immune health.

- **Preparation:** Consume raw, dried, or as juice.

- **Benefits:** Rich in vitamin C; boosts immunity and has antioxidant properties.

- **Safety:** Generally safe; consult a healthcare provider if on certain medications.

189. Olive Leaf

- **Uses:** Antimicrobial, immune support.

- **Preparation:** Brew tea or take as a supplement.

- **Benefits:** Contains oleuropein, which may support immunity and have antimicrobial effects.

- **Safety:** Generally safe; may cause gastrointestinal upset in some individuals.

190. Blackcurrant

- **Uses:** Antioxidant support, respiratory health.

- **Preparation:** Consume raw, as juice, or in supplements.

- **Benefits:** High in vitamin C and antioxidants; supports respiratory health.

- **Safety:** Generally safe; wash thoroughly to avoid pesticide exposure.

191. Saffron

- **Uses:** Mood enhancement, antioxidant support.

- **Preparation:** Use as a spice in cooking or brew tea.

- **Benefits:** May improve mood and has antioxidant properties.

- **Safety:** Generally safe; excessive amounts can cause toxicity.

192. Quinoa

- **Uses:** Nutritional support, gluten-free grain alternative.

- **Preparation:** Cook like rice.

- **Benefits:** High in protein and fiber; suitable for gluten-sensitive individuals.

- **Safety:** Generally safe; consult a healthcare provider for personalized dietary advice.

193. Alfalfa

- **Uses:** Nutritional support, cholesterol regulation.

- **Preparation:** Consume as sprouts or in supplements.

- **Benefits:** Rich in vitamins and minerals; may help lower cholesterol.

- **Safety:** Generally safe; may interact with blood thinners.

194. White Willow Bark

- **Uses:** Pain relief, inflammation.

- **Preparation:** Brew tea or take as a supplement.

- **Benefits:** Contains salicin; may relieve pain and reduce inflammation.

- **Safety:** Generally safe; may cause stomach upset in some individuals.

195. Oregano Oil

- **Uses:** Antimicrobial, respiratory health.

- **Preparation:** Use diluted topically or as a supplement.

- **Benefits:** Antimicrobial properties; may support respiratory health.

- **Safety:** Generally safe; may cause skin irritation if not diluted.

196. Curry Leaves

- **Uses:** Digestive health, blood sugar regulation.

- **Preparation:** Use fresh in cooking or as a powder.

- **Benefits:** May help with digestion and regulate blood sugar levels.

- **Safety:** Generally safe; avoid large amounts.

197. Chia Seeds

- **Uses:** Digestive health, nutritional support.

- **Preparation:** Soak and consume in smoothies or yogurt.

- **Benefits:** High in omega-3s and fiber; promotes digestive health.

- **Safety:** Generally safe; ensure proper hydration to avoid choking.

198. Pine Bark Extract (Pycnogenol)

- **Uses:** Antioxidant support, circulatory health.

- **Preparation:** Take as a supplement.

- **Benefits:** High in antioxidants; may support circulatory health.

- **Safety:** Generally safe; may interact with anticoagulants.

199. Pomegranate

- **Uses:** Antioxidant support, heart health.

- **Preparation:** Consume raw or as juice.

- **Benefits:** High in antioxidants; supports heart health.

- **Safety:** Generally safe; consult a healthcare provider if on medications.

200. Honey

- **Uses:** Soothing sore throat, wound healing.

- **Preparation:** Use raw in teas or as a topical agent.

- **Benefits:** Antimicrobial properties; soothes throat and aids wound healing.

- **Safety:** Generally safe; avoid giving honey to infants under one year.

201. Ashwagandha

- **Uses:** Stress relief, anxiety, and fatigue.

- **Preparation:** Take as a powder, capsule, or tincture.

- **Benefits:** Adaptogen that may help reduce stress and improve energy levels.

- **Safety:** Generally safe; may cause digestive upset in some individuals.

202. Schisandra Berry

- **Uses:** Stress relief, liver health.

- **Preparation:** Brew tea or take as a supplement.

- **Benefits:** May support liver function and enhance physical performance.

- **Safety:** Generally safe; consult a healthcare provider if pregnant.

203. Fennel Seeds

- **Uses:** Digestive health, bloating relief.

- **Preparation:** Brew tea or chew seeds.

- **Benefits:** May alleviate bloating and improve digestion.

- **Safety:** Generally safe; avoid excessive consumption.

204. Moringa

- **Uses:** Nutritional support, energy booster.

- **Preparation:** Consume as a powder in smoothies or as capsules.

- **Benefits:** Rich in vitamins and minerals; may boost energy and nutrition.

- **Safety:** Generally safe; consult a healthcare provider if pregnant.

205. Valerian Root

- **Uses:** Sleep aid, anxiety relief.

- **Preparation:** Brew tea or take as a supplement.

- **Benefits:** May promote relaxation and improve sleep quality.

- **Safety:** Generally safe; may cause drowsiness; avoid operating machinery after use.

206. Cabbage

- **Uses:** Digestive health, skin issues.

- **Preparation:** Eat raw, fermented (sauerkraut), or cooked.

- **Benefits:** High in fiber; may help with digestion and skin conditions.

- **Safety:** Generally safe; may cause gas in some individuals.

207. Bilberry

- **Uses:** Eye health, circulation.

- **Preparation:** Take as a supplement or consume fresh or dried berries.

- **Benefits:** May improve vision and support circulation.

- **Safety:** Generally safe; may interact with blood thinners.

208. Cacao

- **Uses:** Mood enhancement, antioxidant support.

- **Preparation:** Use raw in smoothies or as dark chocolate.

- **Benefits:** Contains flavonoids; may boost mood and provide antioxidant support.

- **Safety:** Generally safe; excessive consumption may lead to caffeine-related side effects.

209. Mustard Seeds

- **Uses:** Digestive health, respiratory support.

- **Preparation:** Use in cooking or brew as tea.

- **Benefits:** May aid digestion and support respiratory health.

- **Safety:** Generally safe; excessive consumption may cause stomach upset.

210. Eleuthero (Siberian Ginseng)

- **Uses:** Energy booster, immune support.

- **Preparation:** Take as a supplement or brew tea.

- **Benefits:** May enhance stamina and immune function.

- **Safety:** Generally safe; consult a healthcare provider if on medications.

211. Lemon Balm

- **Uses:** Anxiety relief, sleep aid.

- **Preparation:** Brew tea from fresh or dried leaves.

- **Benefits:** Calming effects; may help improve sleep quality.

- **Safety:** Generally safe; may cause drowsiness.

212. Gotu Kola

- **Uses:** Cognitive support, wound healing.

- **Preparation:** Consume as a supplement or brew tea.

- **Benefits:** May improve memory and accelerate wound healing.

- **Safety:** Generally safe; may cause skin irritation in some individuals.

213. Black Seed

- **Uses:** Immune support, respiratory health.

- **Preparation:** Consume seeds raw or as oil.

- **Benefits:** Antioxidant properties; may enhance immune function.

- **Safety:** Generally safe; consult a healthcare provider if pregnant.

214. Papaya

- **Uses:** Digestive health, skin care.

- **Preparation:** Eat raw or use in smoothies.

- **Benefits:** Contains enzymes that aid digestion; beneficial for skin.

- **Safety:** Generally safe; excessive consumption may cause digestive upset.

215. Red Clover

- **Uses:** Hormonal balance, menopausal symptoms.

- **Preparation:** Brew tea or take as a supplement.

- **Benefits:** May alleviate menopausal symptoms and support hormonal balance.

- **Safety:** Generally safe; consult a healthcare provider if on hormone therapy.

216. Cumin Seeds

- **Uses:** Digestive health, antioxidant support.

- **Preparation:** Use whole or ground in cooking or brew as tea.

- **Benefits:** May improve digestion and have antioxidant properties.

- **Safety:** Generally safe; avoid excessive amounts.

217. Dulse

- **Uses:** Nutritional support, thyroid health.

- **Preparation:** Eat raw or as a seasoning in meals.

- **Benefits:** Rich in iodine and minerals; supports thyroid function.

- **Safety:** Generally safe; excessive iodine intake may cause thyroid issues.

218. Black Cohosh

- **Uses:** Menopausal symptoms, hormonal balance.

- **Preparation:** Take as a supplement or brew tea.

- **Benefits:** May help alleviate hot flashes and support hormonal balance.

- **Safety:** Consult a healthcare provider if on hormone therapy or pregnant.

219. Coconut Oil

- **Uses:** Skin care, digestive health.

- **Preparation:** Use as cooking oil or apply topically.

- **Benefits:** Antimicrobial properties; promotes skin health and digestion.

- **Safety:** Generally safe; high in saturated fats; moderate consumption recommended.

220. Artichoke

- **Uses:** Digestive health, liver support.

- **Preparation:** Cooked or as a supplement.

- **Benefits:** May aid digestion and support liver function.

- **Safety:** Generally safe; consult a healthcare provider if on diuretics.

221. Red Raspberry Leaf

- **Uses:** Women's health, menstrual relief.

- **Preparation:** Brew tea from dried leaves.

- **Benefits:** May help regulate menstrual cycles and support pregnancy.

- **Safety:** Generally safe; consult a healthcare provider if pregnant.

222. Bay Leaves

- **Uses:** Digestive health, flavoring.

- **Preparation:** Use in cooking or brew as tea.

- **Benefits:** May aid digestion and enhance flavor in dishes.

- **Safety:** Generally safe; avoid consuming whole leaves.

223. Lobelia

- **Uses:** Respiratory health, smoking cessation.

- **Preparation:** Take as a tincture or capsule.

- **Benefits:** May help with respiratory issues and reduce nicotine cravings.

- **Safety:** May cause nausea; consult a healthcare provider before use.

224. Grapefruit Seed Extract

- **Uses:** Antimicrobial, digestive health.

- **Preparation:** Take as a supplement or diluted in water.

- **Benefits:** May support immune function and gut health.

- **Safety:** May interact with medications; consult a healthcare provider.

225. Coconut Milk

- **Uses:** Nutritional support, dairy alternative.

- **Preparation:** Use in cooking or smoothies.

- **Benefits:** Rich in healthy fats; good dairy alternative.

- **Safety:** Generally safe; consult a healthcare provider if on a low-fat diet.

226. Seaweed

- **Uses:** Nutritional support, thyroid health.

- **Preparation:** Use in cooking or supplements.

- **Benefits:** High in iodine and minerals; supports thyroid function.

- **Safety:** Generally safe; excessive iodine intake may cause thyroid issues.

227. Amaranth

- **Uses:** Nutritional support, gluten-free grain.

- **Preparation:** Cook like rice or add to soups.

- **Benefits:** High in protein and fiber; suitable for gluten-sensitive individuals.

- **Safety:** Generally safe; consult a healthcare provider for personalized dietary advice.

228. Black Garlic

- **Uses:** Immune support, heart health.

- **Preparation:** Use in cooking or as a supplement.

- **Benefits:** Contains antioxidants; may support heart health.

- **Safety:** Generally safe; may cause digestive upset in some individuals.

229. Butternut Squash

- **Uses:** Nutritional support, digestive health.

- **Preparation:** Cooked or pureed in soups.

- **Benefits:** High in vitamins and fiber; supports digestion.

- **Safety:** Generally safe; consult a healthcare provider for personalized dietary advice.

230. Poppy Seeds

- **Uses:** Nutritional support, digestive health.

- **Preparation:** Use in cooking or baking.

- **Benefits:** Rich in nutrients; may aid digestion.

- **Safety:** Generally safe; excessive amounts may cause digestive upset.

231. Ginseng

- **Uses:** Energy booster, cognitive support.

- **Preparation:** Take as a supplement or brew tea.

- **Benefits:** May enhance energy levels and cognitive function.

- **Safety:** Generally safe; may interact with medications.

232. Horseradish

- **Uses:** Respiratory health, digestion.

- **Preparation:** Use fresh grated or in sauces.

- **Benefits:** May support respiratory health and digestion.

- **Safety:** Generally safe; excessive amounts can cause gastrointestinal irritation.

233. Cilantro

- **Uses:** Detoxification, digestive health.

- **Preparation:** Use fresh in salads or cooking.

- **Benefits:** May aid in detoxifying heavy metals and improving digestion.

- **Safety:** Generally safe; ensure no allergies to related plants.

234. Flaxseeds

- **Uses:** Digestive health, heart health.

- **Preparation:** Ground in smoothies or oatmeal.

- **Benefits:** High in omega-3 fatty acids and fiber; supports heart health.

- **Safety:** Generally safe; ensure adequate hydration to avoid digestive issues.

235. Parsley

- **Uses:** Digestive health, kidney support.

- **Preparation:** Use fresh in cooking or as tea.

- **Benefits:** May aid digestion and support kidney function.

- **Safety:** Generally safe; excessive amounts can lead to digestive upset.

236. Ginkgo Biloba

- **Uses:** Cognitive support, memory enhancement.

- **Preparation:** Take as a supplement or brew tea.

- **Benefits:** May improve memory and cognitive function.

- **Safety:** Generally safe; may interact with blood thinners.

237. Star Anise

- **Uses:** Digestive health, respiratory support.

- **Preparation:** Use in cooking or brew tea.

- **Benefits:** May relieve digestive issues and respiratory congestion.

- **Safety:** Generally safe; avoid excessive consumption.

238. Nettle

- **Uses:** Allergy relief, nutrient support.
- **Preparation:** Brew tea or consume as a supplement.
- **Benefits:** May alleviate allergy symptoms and is high in nutrients.
- **Safety:** Generally safe; may cause skin irritation if handled fresh.

239. Hawthorn Berries

- **Uses:** Heart health, circulation support.
- **Preparation:** Take as a supplement or brew tea.
- **Benefits:** May support cardiovascular health and circulation.
- **Safety:** Generally safe; consult a healthcare provider if on heart medications.

240. Ceylon Cinnamon

- **Uses:** Blood sugar regulation, anti-inflammatory.
- **Preparation:** Use as a spice in cooking or brew tea.
- **Benefits:** May help regulate blood sugar and reduce inflammation.
- **Safety:** Generally safe; excessive amounts may cause liver issues.

241. Basil

- **Uses:** Digestive health, anti-inflammatory.
- **Preparation:** Use fresh in salads or cooking; brew tea from dried leaves.
- **Benefits:** May reduce inflammation and aid digestion.
- **Safety:** Generally safe; may cause allergic reactions in some individuals.

242. Beetroot

- **Uses:** Blood pressure support, detoxification.
- **Preparation:** Juice or cook and eat.

- **Benefits:** High in nitrates; may help lower blood pressure.

- **Safety:** Generally safe; excessive consumption may cause beeturia (pink urine).

243. Catnip

- **Uses:** Calming effects, digestive health.

- **Preparation:** Brew tea or take as a tincture.

- **Benefits:** May promote relaxation and alleviate digestive issues.

- **Safety:** Generally safe; consult a healthcare provider if pregnant.

244. Comfrey

- **Uses:** Wound healing, inflammation reduction.

- **Preparation:** Use as a topical ointment or salve.

- **Benefits:** May promote wound healing and reduce inflammation.

- **Safety:** Avoid internal use; topical use should be short-term due to potential liver toxicity.

245. Dill

- **Uses:** Digestive aid, anti-inflammatory.

- **Preparation:** Use fresh in cooking or brew tea.

- **Benefits:** May alleviate digestive discomfort and reduce inflammation.

- **Safety:** Generally safe; consult a healthcare provider if pregnant.

246. Elderflower

- **Uses:** Respiratory health, cold relief.

- **Preparation:** Brew tea or use in syrups.

- **Benefits:** May alleviate symptoms of colds and sinusitis.

- **Safety:** Generally safe; may cause allergic reactions in some individuals.

247. Grape Juice

- **Uses:** Heart health, antioxidant support.

- **Preparation:** Drink fresh juice or consume as part of a balanced diet.

- **Benefits:** Rich in antioxidants; may support heart health.

- **Safety:** Generally safe; high sugar content may affect blood sugar levels.

248. Horsetail

- **Uses:** Bone health, hair care.

- **Preparation:** Brew tea or take as a supplement.

- **Benefits:** High in silica; may support bone health and improve hair strength.

- **Safety:** Generally safe; avoid long-term use due to potential toxicity in large amounts.

249. Licorice Root

- **Uses:** Digestive health, respiratory support.

- **Preparation:** Brew tea or take as a supplement.

- **Benefits:** May soothe digestive issues and relieve coughs.

- **Safety:** Long-term use can lead to high blood pressure; consult a healthcare provider.

250. Marshmallow Root

- **Uses:** Digestive health, skin soothing.

- **Preparation:** Brew tea or use in topical preparations.

- **Benefits:** May soothe mucous membranes and alleviate digestive discomfort.

- **Safety:** Generally safe; consult a healthcare provider if on medications.

251. Myrrh

- **Uses:** Oral health, wound healing.

- **Preparation:** Use as an essential oil or in tinctures.

- **Benefits:** Antimicrobial properties; may promote oral health and wound healing.

- **Safety:** Generally safe; avoid internal use in large amounts.

252. Neem

- **Uses:** Skin care, oral health.

- **Preparation:** Use as a paste, oil, or supplement.

- **Benefits:** Antibacterial and antifungal; may promote healthy skin.

- **Safety:** Consult a healthcare provider if pregnant; may cause allergic reactions.

253. Nutmeg

- **Uses:** Digestive aid, sleep support.

- **Preparation:** Use as a spice in cooking or brew tea.

- **Benefits:** May relieve digestive issues and promote relaxation.

- **Safety:** Excessive consumption can be toxic; use in moderation.

254. Passionflower

- **Uses:** Anxiety relief, sleep aid.

- **Preparation:** Brew tea or take as a supplement.

- **Benefits:** May help reduce anxiety and improve sleep quality.

- **Safety:** Generally safe; may cause drowsiness; avoid driving after use.

255. Pineapple

- **Uses:** Digestive health, inflammation reduction.

- **Preparation:** Eat fresh or juice.

- **Benefits:** Contains bromelain, which may aid digestion and reduce inflammation.

- **Safety:** Generally safe; may cause allergic reactions in sensitive individuals.

256. Plantain

- **Uses:** Wound healing, respiratory support.

- **Preparation:** Use leaves topically or brew tea.

- **Benefits:** May promote wound healing and relieve coughs.

- **Safety:** Generally safe; consult a healthcare provider if pregnant.

257. Rosemary

- **Uses:** Cognitive support, digestive health.

- **Preparation:** Use fresh or dried in cooking or brew tea.

- **Benefits:** May enhance memory and aid digestion.

- **Safety:** Generally safe; excessive amounts can cause digestive upset.

258. Saffron

- **Uses:** Mood enhancement, menstrual relief.

- **Preparation:** Use as a spice or brew tea.

- **Benefits:** May improve mood and alleviate menstrual symptoms.

- **Safety:** Generally safe; excessive consumption can cause toxicity.

259. Sage

- **Uses:** Digestive health, respiratory support.

- **Preparation:** Use fresh or dried in cooking or brew tea.

- **Benefits:** May alleviate digestive issues and promote respiratory health.

- **Safety:** Generally safe; excessive consumption may cause digestive upset.

260. Shatavari

- **Uses:** Women's health, hormonal balance.

- **Preparation:** Take as a powder or supplement.

- **Benefits:** May support hormonal balance and reproductive health.

- **Safety:** Generally safe; consult a healthcare provider if pregnant.

261. Slippery Elm

- **Uses:** Digestive health, throat soothing.

- **Preparation:** Brew tea or take as a lozenge.

- **Benefits:** May soothe the digestive tract and relieve throat irritation.

- **Safety:** Generally safe; may interfere with medication absorption.

262. Spearmint

- **Uses:** Digestive aid, respiratory health.

- **Preparation:** Brew tea or use fresh in dishes.

- **Benefits:** May relieve digestive discomfort and promote respiratory health.

- **Safety:** Generally safe; may cause allergic reactions in some individuals.

263. Thyme

- **Uses:** Respiratory health, antiseptic.

- **Preparation:** Use fresh or dried in cooking or brew tea.

- **Benefits:** Antimicrobial properties; may alleviate respiratory issues.

- **Safety:** Generally safe; may cause allergic reactions in sensitive individuals.

264. Turmeric

- **Uses:** Anti-inflammatory, pain relief.

- **Preparation:** Use fresh or as a spice in cooking; take as a supplement.

- **Benefits:** Contains curcumin, which may reduce inflammation and pain.

- **Safety:** Generally safe; excessive consumption may cause digestive upset.

265. Wheatgrass

- **Uses:** Nutritional support, detoxification.

- **Preparation:** Juice or add to smoothies.

- **Benefits:** Rich in vitamins and antioxidants; may aid in detoxification.

- **Safety:** Generally safe; consult a healthcare provider if allergic to grass.

266. Yarrow

- **Uses:** Wound healing, digestive support.

- **Preparation:** Use in teas or topical applications.

- **Benefits:** May promote wound healing and alleviate digestive issues.

- **Safety:** Generally safe; may cause allergic reactions in some individuals.

267. Zinc

- **Uses:** Immune support, wound healing.

- **Preparation:** Take as a supplement or eat zinc-rich foods.

- **Benefits:** Essential for immune function and healing.

- **Safety:** Excessive intake can cause nausea; follow dosage guidelines.

268. Calendula

- **Uses:** Skin healing, inflammation reduction.

- **Preparation:** Use as an oil, salve, or tea.

- **Benefits:** Antimicrobial properties; may promote skin healing.

- **Safety:** Generally safe; may cause allergic reactions in sensitive individuals.

269. Borage

- **Uses:** Skin health, anti-inflammatory.
- **Preparation:** Use oil topically or as a supplement.
- **Benefits:** May help with skin conditions and reduce inflammation.
- **Safety:** Consult a healthcare provider if pregnant; avoid excessive consumption.

270. Cloves

- **Uses:** Dental care, digestive health.
- **Preparation:** Use as a spice in cooking or brew tea.
- **Benefits:** May alleviate dental pain and support digestion.
- **Safety:** Generally safe; excessive consumption can be toxic.

271. Orange Peel

- **Uses:** Digestive health, respiratory support.
- **Preparation:** Use dried peel in teas or cooking.
- **Benefits:** May aid digestion and promote respiratory health.
- **Safety:** Generally safe; consult a healthcare provider if allergic.

272. Bilberry Leaf

- **Uses:** Blood sugar regulation, eye health.
- **Preparation:** Brew tea from dried leaves.
- **Benefits:** May help regulate blood sugar and support vision.
- **Safety:** Generally safe; consult a healthcare provider if pregnant.

273. Catuaba

- **Uses:** Libido enhancement, fatigue relief.

- **Preparation:** Brew tea from bark or take as a supplement.

- **Benefits:** Traditionally used as an aphrodisiac; may boost energy.

- **Safety:** Generally safe; consult a healthcare provider if pregnant.

274. Dandelion Greens

- **Uses:** Liver support, digestive aid.

- **Preparation:** Use fresh in salads or brew tea.

- **Benefits:** May support liver function and improve digestion.

- **Safety:** Generally safe; may cause allergic reactions in some individuals

275. Burdock Root

- **Uses:** Detoxification, skin health.

- **Preparation:** Brew tea or take as a tincture.

- **Benefits:** May help purify the blood and improve skin conditions.

- **Safety:** Generally safe; consult a healthcare provider if pregnant.

276. Blue Vervain

- **Uses:** Anxiety relief, digestive aid.

- **Preparation:** Brew tea or take as a tincture.

- **Benefits:** May reduce anxiety and soothe digestive issues.

- **Safety:** Generally safe; avoid use during pregnancy.

277. Gotu Kola

- **Uses:** Cognitive support, skin health.

- **Preparation:** Brew tea or take as a supplement.

- **Benefits:** May enhance mental clarity and promote skin healing.

- **Safety:** Generally safe; consult a healthcare provider if pregnant.

278. Quassia Bark

- **Uses:** Digestive health, parasite cleansing.

- **Preparation:** Brew tea or take as a tincture.

- **Benefits:** May stimulate digestion and help eliminate parasites.

- **Safety:** Use in moderation; avoid during pregnancy.

279. Red Clover

- **Uses:** Hormone balance, skin health.

- **Preparation:** Brew tea or take as a tincture.

- **Benefits:** Contains phytoestrogens; may support hormonal balance.

- **Safety:** Avoid if pregnant or on hormone-sensitive medications.

280. Black Walnut

- **Uses:** Parasite cleansing, skin health.

- **Preparation:** Use as a tincture or topical application.

- **Benefits:** Antimicrobial properties; may help cleanse the body.

- **Safety:** Avoid if pregnant; long-term use not recommended.

281. Shepherd's Purse

- **Uses:** Bleeding control, menstrual support.

- **Preparation:** Brew tea or use as a tincture.

- **Benefits:** Traditionally used to help reduce bleeding.

- **Safety:** Avoid during pregnancy.

282. Agrimony

- **Uses:** Digestive health, skin healing.

- **Preparation:** Brew tea or apply topically.

- **Benefits:** May soothe digestive issues and aid skin healing.

- **Safety:** Generally safe; avoid if on blood-thinning medication.

283. Yellow Dock

- **Uses:** Liver support, digestive health.

- **Preparation:** Brew tea or use as a tincture.

- **Benefits:** May support liver function and improve digestion.

- **Safety:** May cause mild digestive upset in large amounts.

284. Red Raspberry Leaf

- **Uses:** Women's reproductive health, menstrual support.

- **Preparation:** Brew tea.

- **Benefits:** May tone the uterus and support pregnancy.

- **Safety:** Consult a healthcare provider if pregnant.

285. Wormwood

- **Uses:** Parasite cleansing, digestive health.

- **Preparation:** Brew tea or use as a tincture.

- **Benefits:** Traditionally used to eliminate parasites.

- **Safety:** Avoid in pregnancy; do not use long-term.

286. Cardamom

- **Uses:** Digestive health, respiratory support.

- **Preparation:** Use as a spice or brew tea.

- **Benefits:** May soothe indigestion and support respiratory health.

- **Safety:** Generally safe in culinary amounts.

287. Goldenseal

- **Uses:** Immune support, digestive health.

- **Preparation:** Brew tea or use as a tincture.

- **Benefits:** Contains berberine; may boost immunity.

- **Safety:** Avoid if pregnant or breastfeeding; may interact with medications.

288. Maca Root

- **Uses:** Energy, hormonal balance.

- **Preparation:** Take as a powder or supplement.

- **Benefits:** May enhance energy and support hormone balance.

- **Safety:** Generally safe; consult if thyroid-sensitive.

289. Rhodiola

- **Uses:** Stress relief, energy support.

- **Preparation:** Brew tea or take as a supplement.

- **Benefits:** Adaptogen; may reduce stress and fatigue.

- **Safety:** Avoid high doses; may cause jitteriness in sensitive individuals.

290. Skullcap

- **Uses:** Anxiety relief, nerve support.

- **Preparation:** Brew tea or take as a tincture.

- **Benefits:** May promote relaxation and support the nervous system.

- **Safety:** Generally safe; may cause drowsiness.

291. Schisandra

- **Uses:** Stress relief, liver support.

- **Preparation:** Brew tea or take as a supplement.

- **Benefits:** Adaptogen; may support stress resilience and liver health.

- **Safety:** Generally safe; avoid if pregnant.

292. Gymnema Sylvestre

- **Uses:** Blood sugar regulation, appetite control.

- **Preparation:** Take as a supplement.

- **Benefits:** May help regulate blood sugar levels.

- **Safety:** Consult a healthcare provider if diabetic.

293. Horny Goat Weed

- **Uses:** Libido enhancement, energy support.

- **Preparation:** Take as a supplement.

- **Benefits:** May enhance libido and reduce fatigue.

- **Safety:** Consult a healthcare provider if on medication.

294. Buchu

- **Uses:** Urinary tract health, kidney support.

- **Preparation:** Brew tea.

- **Benefits:** Traditionally used to support urinary health.

- **Safety:** Avoid if pregnant; consult a healthcare provider for long-term use.

295. Fenugreek

- **Uses:** Digestive health, lactation support.

- **Preparation:** Brew tea or take as a supplement.

- **Benefits:** May support digestion and milk production in breastfeeding women.

- **Safety:** Avoid if pregnant.

296. Uva Ursi

- **Uses:** Urinary health, bladder support.

- **Preparation:** Brew tea or take as a supplement.

- **Benefits:** May help with urinary tract infections.

- **Safety:** Avoid if pregnant; short-term use recommended.

297. Damiana

- **Uses:** Mood enhancement, libido support.

- **Preparation:** Brew tea or take as a supplement.

- **Benefits:** Traditionally used to support mood and libido.

- **Safety:** Generally safe; consult a healthcare provider if pregnant.

298. Sea Buckthorn

- **Uses:** Skin health, immune support.

- **Preparation:** Take as a supplement or use topically.

- **Benefits:** High in vitamins; may support skin and immune health.

- **Safety:** Generally safe; avoid if allergic to berries.

299. Copaiba

- **Uses:** Inflammation relief, pain support.

- **Preparation:** Use as an essential oil or topical application.

- **Benefits:** Anti-inflammatory; may help relieve pain.

- **Safety:** Avoid internal use without professional guidance.

300. Artemisia Annua (Sweet Wormwood)

- **Uses:** Immune support, parasite cleansing.

- **Preparation:** Brew tea or take as a supplement.

- **Benefits:** Traditionally used for immune health and parasites.

- **Safety:** Avoid if pregnant; do not use long-term.

301. Barberry

- **Uses:** Digestive health, immune support.

- **Preparation:** Brew tea or use as a tincture.

- **Benefits:** Contains berberine; may support digestion and immunity.

- **Safety:** Avoid if pregnant; may interact with medications.

302. Jiaogulan

- **Uses:** Stress relief, immune support.

- **Preparation:** Brew tea.

- **Benefits:** Adaptogen; may reduce stress and support immunity.

- **Safety:** Generally safe; avoid if pregnant.

303. Andrographis

- **Uses:** Immune support, anti-inflammatory.

- **Preparation:** Take as a supplement or brew tea.

- **Benefits:** May enhance immunity and reduce inflammation.

- **Safety:** Avoid in pregnancy; consult a healthcare provider for prolonged use.

304. Stone Root

- **Uses:** Urinary health, vein support.

- **Preparation:** Brew tea or take as a tincture.

- **Benefits:** May support urinary tract and vascular health.

- **Safety:** Generally safe; consult if on blood-thinning medication.

305. Coptis (Chinese Goldthread)

- **Uses:** Digestive health, immune support.

- **Preparation:** Take as a supplement.

- **Benefits:** Contains berberine; may support digestion and immunity.

- **Safety:** Avoid if pregnant; consult for prolonged use.

306. Ashoka

- **Uses:** Women's reproductive health.

- **Preparation:** Take as a supplement.

- **Benefits:** Traditionally used to support menstrual health.

- **Safety:** Generally safe; consult a healthcare provider if pregnant.

307. Blue Lotus

- **Uses:** Relaxation, sleep support.

- **Preparation:** Brew tea or take as a tincture.

- **Benefits:** May promote relaxation and aid sleep.

- **Safety:** Avoid if pregnant; consult for appropriate use.

308. Bacopa Monnieri

- **Uses:** Cognitive support, memory enhancement.

- **Preparation:** Take as a supplement.

- **Benefits:** May support memory and cognitive function.

- **Safety:** Consult if on medications; avoid during pregnancy.

309. Guayusa

- **Uses:** Energy, focus.

- **Preparation:** Brew tea.

- **Benefits:** Contains caffeine; may enhance energy and focus.

- **Safety:** Avoid if caffeine-sensitive or pregnant.

310. Oregon Grape

- **Uses:** Immune support, skin health.

- **Preparation:** Brew tea or take as a tincture.

- **Benefits:** Contains berberine; may support immunity and skin.

- **Safety:** Avoid if pregnant; consult if on medication.

311. Galangal

- **Uses:** Digestive health, inflammation relief.

- **Preparation:** Brew tea or use as a spice in cooking.

- **Benefits:** Similar to ginger; may reduce nausea and inflammation.

- **Safety:** Generally safe in culinary amounts; avoid high doses.

312. Lemon Balm

- **Uses:** Anxiety relief, digestive health.

- **Preparation:** Brew tea or use in tincture form.

- **Benefits:** May promote relaxation and soothe digestion.

- **Safety:** Safe in moderation; may interact with thyroid medications.

313. Juniper Berry

- **Uses:** Urinary health, inflammation.

- **Preparation:** Brew tea or use as a spice.

- **Benefits:** May aid in urinary health and reduce inflammation.

- **Safety:** Avoid if pregnant or have kidney issues.

314. Devil's Claw

- **Uses:** Pain relief, joint health.

- **Preparation:** Take as a supplement or brew tea.

- **Benefits:** Anti-inflammatory; may relieve joint pain.

- **Safety:** Avoid if pregnant or have gastrointestinal issues.

315. Oregon Grape Root

- **Uses:** Skin health, digestive support.

- **Preparation:** Use as a tincture or brew tea.

- **Benefits:** Contains berberine; may improve skin and digestion.

- **Safety:** Avoid in pregnancy; consult if on medication.

316. Solomon's Seal

- **Uses:** Joint health, injury recovery.

- **Preparation:** Use as a tincture or tea.

- **Benefits:** May support joint and tendon health.

- **Safety:** Generally safe; avoid long-term use without professional guidance.

317. Wood Betony

- **Uses:** Nervous system health, headaches.

- **Preparation:** Brew tea.

- **Benefits:** Traditionally used to calm the nerves and relieve headaches.

- **Safety:** Generally safe in moderation.

318. Valerian Root

- **Uses:** Sleep support, anxiety relief.

- **Preparation:** Brew tea or take as a tincture.

- **Benefits:** May improve sleep quality and reduce anxiety.

- **Safety:** Avoid in large doses; may cause drowsiness.

319. Shatavari

- **Uses:** Women's health, reproductive support.

- **Preparation:** Take as a supplement or brew tea.

- **Benefits:** Adaptogen; supports hormonal balance in women.

- **Safety:** Generally safe; consult if pregnant.

320. California Poppy

- **Uses:** Sleep support, pain relief.

- **Preparation:** Brew tea or take as a tincture.

- **Benefits:** May promote relaxation and relieve mild pain.

- **Safety:** Avoid if pregnant; may cause mild drowsiness.

321. Sassafras

- **Uses:** Respiratory health, digestive support.

- **Preparation:** Brew tea.

- **Benefits:** Traditionally used for respiratory support.

- **Safety:** Use in moderation; high doses may be toxic.

322. Celery Seed

- **Uses:** Joint health, inflammation relief.

- **Preparation:** Brew tea or use as a spice.

- **Benefits:** May reduce inflammation and improve joint health.

- **Safety:** Avoid if pregnant; consult for prolonged use.

323. Eyebright

- **Uses:** Eye health, sinus relief.

- **Preparation:** Brew tea or use in eyewashes.

- **Benefits:** May support eye health and reduce sinus issues.

- **Safety:** Consult for use in eyewashes; avoid if allergic.

324. Linden Flower

- **Uses:** Anxiety relief, sleep support.

- **Preparation:** Brew tea.

- **Benefits:** May reduce anxiety and promote restful sleep.

- **Safety:** Generally safe; avoid in pregnancy.

325. Self-Heal (Prunella Vulgaris)

- **Uses:** Skin health, immune support.

- **Preparation:** Brew tea or apply topically.

- **Benefits:** Traditionally used for wound healing and immune support.

- **Safety:** Generally safe; avoid if allergic.

326. Lady's Mantle

- **Uses:** Menstrual support, skin health.

- **Preparation:** Brew tea.

- **Benefits:** Traditionally used for menstrual health and wound care.

- **Safety:** Avoid if pregnant; may cause mild digestive upset.

327. Wild Yam

- **Uses:** Hormone balance, menstrual support.

- **Preparation:** Brew tea or take as a tincture.

- **Benefits:** May support hormonal health in women.

- **Safety:** Avoid in pregnancy; consult if on hormone medications.

328. Yarrow

- **Uses:** Wound healing, fever relief.

- **Preparation:** Brew tea or apply topically.

- **Benefits:** May support wound healing and reduce fever.

- **Safety:** Avoid if pregnant; may interact with blood-thinning medications.

329. Bilberry

- **Uses:** Eye health, circulation.

- **Preparation:** Brew tea or take as a supplement.

- **Benefits:** High in antioxidants; may support vision and circulation.

- **Safety:** Generally safe; consult if on blood-thinners.

330. Coltsfoot

- **Uses:** Respiratory health, cough relief.

- **Preparation:** Brew tea.

- **Benefits:** Traditionally used to soothe coughs and respiratory issues.

- **Safety:** Use in moderation; long-term use not recommended.

331. Licorice Root

- **Uses:** Digestive health, respiratory support.

- **Preparation:** Brew tea or use as a tincture.

- **Benefits:** May soothe the digestive tract and respiratory system.

- **Safety:** Avoid in high doses or if hypertensive.

332. Marshmallow Root

- **Uses:** Digestive health, sore throat relief.

- **Preparation:** Brew tea or make a poultice.

- **Benefits:** Soothing to mucous membranes; may relieve sore throat.

- **Safety:** Generally safe; consult if diabetic.

333. Elderflower

- **Uses:** Cold and flu relief, allergy support.

- **Preparation:** Brew tea or make syrup.

- **Benefits:** May reduce cold symptoms and support respiratory health.

- **Safety:** Avoid unripe berries; may cause digestive upset.

334. Holy Basil (Tulsi)

- **Uses:** Stress relief, immune support.

- **Preparation:** Brew tea or take as a supplement.

- **Benefits:** Adaptogen; may support stress resilience and immunity.

- **Safety:** Generally safe; avoid in pregnancy.

335. White Willow Bark

- **Uses:** Pain relief, inflammation.

- **Preparation:** Brew tea or take as a supplement.

- **Benefits:** Natural source of salicin; may relieve pain.

- **Safety:** Avoid if allergic to aspirin or on blood-thinners.

336. Motherwort

- **Uses:** Heart health, anxiety relief.

- **Preparation:** Brew tea or take as a tincture.

- **Benefits:** May support heart health and reduce anxiety.

- **Safety:** Avoid in pregnancy; consult if on medication.

337. Slippery Elm

- **Uses:** Digestive health, sore throat relief.

- **Preparation:** Brew tea or take as a lozenge.

- **Benefits:** Soothing to the digestive and respiratory tracts.

- **Safety:** Generally safe; avoid if pregnant.

338. Peppermint

- **Uses:** Digestive health, headache relief.

- **Preparation:** Brew tea or use as an essential oil.

- **Benefits:** May relieve digestive discomfort and tension headaches.

- **Safety:** Avoid peppermint oil near children's faces.

339. Dandelion Root

- **Uses:** Liver support, digestion.

- **Preparation:** Brew tea or use in tinctures.

- **Benefits:** May support liver health and digestion.

- **Safety:** Generally safe; avoid if allergic to daisies.

340. Sage

- **Uses:** Memory support, digestive health.

- **Preparation:** Brew tea or use in cooking.

- **Benefits:** May improve memory and soothe digestion.

- **Safety:** Avoid high doses if pregnant.

341. Nettle

- **Uses:** Allergy support, iron source.

- **Preparation:** Brew tea or cook as greens.

- **Benefits:** Nutrient-rich; may help with allergies.

- **Safety:** Use gloves when handling fresh nettles.

342. Thyme

- **Uses:** Respiratory health, digestive support.

- **Preparation:** Brew tea or use as a seasoning.

- **Benefits:** Antimicrobial; may aid in respiratory issues.

- **Safety:** Safe in culinary amounts.

343. Parsley

- **Uses:** Kidney health, digestion.

- **Preparation:** Use fresh or brew tea.

- **Benefits:** High in vitamins; may support kidney health.

- **Safety:** Avoid large amounts if pregnant.

344. Angelica Root

- **Uses:** Digestive health, stress relief.

- **Preparation:** Brew tea or take as a tincture.

- **Benefits:** May soothe digestion and relieve stress.

- **Safety:** Avoid in pregnancy; may increase sun sensitivity.

345. Bay Leaf

- **Uses:** Digestion, respiratory support.

- **Preparation:** Use in cooking or brew tea.

- **Benefits:** May support digestion and respiratory health.

- **Safety:** Remove whole leaves before consuming dishes.

346. Horsetail

- **Uses:** Bone health, hair and nail support.

- **Preparation:** Brew tea.

- **Benefits:** Rich in silica; may support bone and nail health.

- **Safety:** Avoid if you have kidney disease.

347. Aloe Vera

- **Uses:** Skin health, digestive support.

- **Preparation:** Apply gel or drink juice.

- **Benefits:** Soothing to skin and digestive tract.

- **Safety:** Consult for internal use; may cause digestive upset.

348. Chicory Root

- **Uses:** Digestive health, prebiotic.

- **Preparation:** Brew tea or add to coffee.

- **Benefits:** Prebiotic fiber; may support gut health.

- **Safety:** Generally safe; avoid in pregnancy.

349. Feverfew

- **Uses:** Migraine relief, inflammation.

- **Preparation:** Brew tea or take as a supplement.

- **Benefits:** May reduce migraine frequency.

- **Safety:** Avoid in pregnancy; may interact with blood-thinners.

350. Gotu Kola

- **Uses:** Mental clarity, skin health.

- **Preparation:** Brew tea or use in skincare.

- **Benefits:** May improve cognitive function and support skin.

- **Safety:** Avoid high doses; consult if on medication.

351. Horehound

- **Uses:** Cough relief, digestive aid.

- **Preparation:** Brew tea or make cough syrup.

- **Benefits:** Known for its expectorant properties; may ease respiratory congestion.

- **Safety:** Generally safe, but avoid during pregnancy.

352. Agrimony

- **Uses:** Digestive health, skin irritation.

- **Preparation:** Brew tea or apply as a poultice.

- **Benefits:** May aid digestion and soothe minor skin irritations.

- **Safety:** Avoid if you have liver disease.

353. Mugwort

- **Uses:** Digestive support, dream enhancement.

- **Preparation:** Brew tea or use as incense.

- **Benefits:** May promote digestion and vivid dreams.

- **Safety:** Avoid in pregnancy; may cause allergic reactions.

354. Elecampane

- **Uses:** Respiratory health, cough relief.

- **Preparation:** Brew tea or make syrup.

- **Benefits:** Traditionally used to ease respiratory issues and coughs.

- **Safety:** Avoid in large doses; consult if pregnant.

355. Skullcap

- **Uses:** Anxiety relief, nervous system support.

- **Preparation:** Brew tea or take as tincture.

- **Benefits:** May calm nerves and promote relaxation.

- **Safety:** Safe in moderation; consult for long-term use.

356. Coltsfoot

- **Uses:** Respiratory health, cough relief.

- **Preparation:** Brew tea.

- **Benefits:** Soothes coughs and respiratory issues.

- **Safety:** Avoid prolonged use; may have liver toxicity risks.

357. Hyssop

- **Uses:** Respiratory support, immune boost.

- **Preparation:** Brew tea or make tincture.

- **Benefits:** May aid in respiratory and immune health.

- **Safety:** Avoid in pregnancy; consult if on medications.

358. Cleavers

- **Uses:** Lymphatic system health, skin health.

- **Preparation:** Brew tea or use in a tincture.

- **Benefits:** Supports the lymphatic system and aids in detox.

- **Safety:** Generally safe in moderation.

359. Butcher's Broom

- **Uses:** Circulatory health, vein support.

- **Preparation:** Brew tea or take in capsules.

- **Benefits:** May help with varicose veins and improve circulation.

- **Safety:** Avoid in pregnancy; consult for high blood pressure.

360. Plantain

- **Uses:** Skin health, digestive aid.

- **Preparation:** Brew tea or apply as a poultice.

- **Benefits:** Helps with skin irritation and digestion.

- **Safety:** Generally safe; avoid if allergic.

361. Gravel Root

- **Uses:** Kidney health, urinary tract support.

- **Preparation:** Brew tea or take as a tincture.

- **Benefits:** Traditionally used for urinary health.

- **Safety:** Avoid in pregnancy; consult for prolonged use.

362. Yellow Dock

- **Uses:** Liver health, skin support.

- **Preparation:** Brew tea or take as a tincture.

- **Benefits:** May support liver function and improve skin health.

- **Safety:** Avoid if pregnant; may have laxative effects.

363. Blue Vervain

- **Uses:** Anxiety relief, nervous system support.
- **Preparation:** Brew tea or take as a tincture.
- **Benefits:** May promote relaxation and reduce anxiety.
- **Safety:** Generally safe; consult if pregnant.

364. Comfrey

- **Uses:** Wound healing, bone health.
- **Preparation:** Apply topically; avoid internal use.
- **Benefits:** Known as a "knit bone" herb; may support healing of wounds and bones.
- **Safety:** External use only; avoid on open wounds.

365. Hops

- **Uses:** Sleep support, digestive aid.
- **Preparation:** Brew tea or use in tinctures.
- **Benefits:** May promote relaxation and improve sleep quality.
- **Safety:** Avoid in pregnancy; may cause drowsiness.

366. Meadowsweet

- **Uses:** Pain relief, digestive health.
- **Preparation:** Brew tea.
- **Benefits:** Natural source of salicin; may aid in pain relief.
- **Safety:** Avoid if allergic to aspirin.

367. Horehound

- **Uses:** Respiratory health, digestive aid.
- **Preparation:** Brew tea or make cough syrup.

- **Benefits:** Expectorant; may relieve respiratory congestion.

- **Safety:** Avoid in pregnancy; consult for prolonged use.

368. Pleurisy Root

- **Uses:** Respiratory support, cough relief.

- **Preparation:** Brew tea.

- **Benefits:** Traditionally used to support lung health.

- **Safety:** Avoid in pregnancy; consult for prolonged use.

369. Blessed Thistle

- **Uses:** Digestive health, liver support.

- **Preparation:** Brew tea.

- **Benefits:** Traditionally used for digestive and liver support.

- **Safety:** Avoid if pregnant or breastfeeding.

370. Anise

- **Uses:** Digestive health, respiratory health.

- **Preparation:** Brew tea or use as a spice.

- **Benefits:** May help with digestion and respiratory issues.

- **Safety:** Avoid high doses; consult if pregnant.

371. Parsley Root

- **Uses:** Kidney health, digestion.

- **Preparation:** Brew tea or use in cooking.

- **Benefits:** May support kidney health and aid digestion.

- **Safety:** Avoid in large amounts during pregnancy.

372. Alfalfa

- **Uses:** Nutrient boost, hormone support.

- **Preparation:** Brew tea or add sprouts to salads.

- **Benefits:** High in nutrients; may support hormone balance.

- **Safety:** Avoid if you have autoimmune conditions.

373. Caraway Seed

- **Uses:** Digestive aid, respiratory health.

- **Preparation:** Brew tea or use as a spice.

- **Benefits:** May soothe digestive discomfort.

- **Safety:** Generally safe in culinary amounts.

374. Bee Balm

- **Uses:** Respiratory health, digestive aid.

- **Preparation:** Brew tea or use topically.

- **Benefits:** Antimicrobial; may aid respiratory and digestive health.

- **Safety:** Generally safe; avoid if allergic.

375. Prickly Ash

- **Uses:** Circulation, pain relief.

- **Preparation:** Brew tea or take as a tincture.

- **Benefits:** Traditionally used to improve circulation.

- **Safety:** Avoid in pregnancy; consult for long-term use.

376. Reishi Mushroom

- **Uses:** Immune support, stress resilience.

- **Preparation:** Brew tea or take as a supplement.

- **Benefits:** Adaptogen; may support immune health.

- **Safety:** Generally safe; consult if on immunosuppressants.

377. Lobelia

- **Uses:** Respiratory health, muscle relaxation.

- **Preparation:** Brew tea or use in tinctures.

- **Benefits:** May relieve respiratory issues and relax muscles.

- **Safety:** Avoid high doses; may cause nausea.

378. Wintergreen

- **Uses:** Pain relief, inflammation.

- **Preparation:** Use topically or brew tea in moderation.

- **Benefits:** Natural source of methyl salicylate; may relieve pain.

- **Safety:** Avoid internal use; toxic in high doses.

379. Bee Pollen

- **Uses:** Nutrient support, allergy relief.

- **Preparation:** Add to smoothies or cereal.

- **Benefits:** Nutrient-dense; may support immune health.

- **Safety:** Avoid if allergic to pollen.

380. Fennel Seed

- **Uses:** Digestive health, respiratory support.

- **Preparation:** Brew tea or use in cooking.

- **Benefits:** Soothes digestion; may ease respiratory issues.

- **Safety:** Generally safe; avoid in high doses during pregnancy.

381. Passionflower

- **Uses:** Anxiety relief, sleep aid.
- **Preparation:** Brew tea or take as tincture.
- **Benefits:** May promote relaxation and reduce anxiety.
- **Safety:** May cause drowsiness; avoid in pregnancy.

382. Mallow

- **Uses:** Digestive health, skin soothing.
- **Preparation:** Brew tea or apply topically.
- **Benefits:** Soothes mucous membranes and irritated skin.
- **Safety:** Generally safe; consult for extended use.

383. Horehound

- **Uses:** Cough relief, digestive health.
- **Preparation:** Brew tea or make cough syrup.
- **Benefits:** Traditionally used for respiratory issues.
- **Safety:** Avoid in pregnancy.

384. Sweet Clover

- **Uses:** Circulation, blood health.
- **Preparation:** Brew tea or use in tinctures.
- **Benefits:** May improve circulation and support vein health.
- **Safety:** Avoid in high doses; contains coumarin.

385. Gotu Kola

- **Uses:** Cognitive support, skin health.
- **Preparation:** Brew tea or use in skincare.

- **Benefits:** May improve memory and support skin.

- **Safety:** Avoid high doses; consult if on medications.

386. Yarrow

- **Uses:** Wound healing, fever relief.

- **Preparation:** Brew tea or apply topically.

- **Benefits:** May support healing and reduce fever.

- **Safety:** Avoid if pregnant; may interact with blood-thinning medications

387. Fo-Ti

- **Uses:** Hair health, longevity.

- **Preparation:** Brew tea or take as a supplement.

- **Benefits:** May support hair growth and overall vitality.

- **Safety:** Consult for prolonged use; may cause digestive upset.

388. Wormwood

- **Uses:** Digestive support, parasitic infections.

- **Preparation:** Brew tea or take as a tincture.

- **Benefits:** Traditionally used to combat digestive parasites and promote digestion.

- **Safety:** Avoid in pregnancy; toxic in high doses.

389. Valerian Root

- **Uses:** Sleep aid, relaxation.

- **Preparation:** Brew tea or take in capsule form.

- **Benefits:** Known for its calming effects; may improve sleep quality.

- **Safety:** May cause drowsiness; avoid long-term use.

390. Bayberry

- **Uses:** Respiratory health, digestive support.

- **Preparation:** Brew tea or make a poultice.

- **Benefits:** May relieve congestion and support digestion.

- **Safety:** Avoid in large doses; may cause digestive upset.

391. Lady's Mantle

- **Uses:** Menstrual support, wound healing.

- **Preparation:** Brew tea or apply topically.

- **Benefits:** Traditionally used to ease menstrual symptoms and promote skin healing.

- **Safety:** Avoid in pregnancy.

392. Myrrh

- **Uses:** Oral health, immune support.

- **Preparation:** Use in tinctures or mouthwash.

- **Benefits:** Antimicrobial properties; supports oral health.

- **Safety:** Avoid in pregnancy; consult if on medication.

393. Buchu

- **Uses:** Urinary health, kidney support.

- **Preparation:** Brew tea or take in tincture.

- **Benefits:** May relieve urinary tract discomfort and support kidney function.

- **Safety:** Avoid in pregnancy and consult for prolonged use.

394. Gravelroot

- **Uses:** Kidney support, urinary health.

- **Preparation:** Brew tea or use in tincture.

- **Benefits:** Supports urinary health; traditionally used for kidney stones.

- **Safety:** Avoid in pregnancy; consult if on medication.

395. Eleuthero (Siberian Ginseng)

- **Uses:** Energy, immune support.

- **Preparation:** Brew tea or take as a supplement.

- **Benefits:** Adaptogen that may enhance energy and immune resilience.

- **Safety:** Avoid in pregnancy; consult if on medications.

396. Chaga Mushroom

- **Uses:** Immune support, antioxidant boost.

- **Preparation:** Brew as a tea or take as a supplement.

- **Benefits:** Known for immune support and high antioxidant content.

- **Safety:** Generally safe; consult if on blood-thinning medications.

397. Horsetail

- **Uses:** Bone health, skin and hair support.

- **Preparation:** Brew tea or use in a poultice.

- **Benefits:** High in silica, supporting hair, skin, and nails.

- **Safety:** Avoid in large doses; consult if you have kidney issues.

398. Spikenard

- **Uses:** Respiratory health, skin health.

- **Preparation:** Use in aromatherapy or apply topically.

- **Benefits:** Known for its calming effects and respiratory support.

- **Safety:** Generally safe; avoid if allergic.

399. Prunella (Self-Heal)

- **Uses:** Wound healing, immune support.

- **Preparation:** Brew tea or apply topically.

- **Benefits:** Known for wound healing and immune support.

- **Safety:** Generally safe; avoid if allergic.

400. Linden Flower

- **Uses:** Relaxation, respiratory health.

- **Preparation:** Brew tea.

- **Benefits:** May help with relaxation and ease respiratory issues.

- **Safety:** Generally safe; avoid in large doses.

401. Slippery Elm

- **Uses:** Digestive health, throat soothing.

- **Preparation:** Brew tea or take lozenges.

- **Benefits:** Soothes throat and digestive tract.

- **Safety:** Generally safe; avoid if pregnant.

402. White Oak Bark

- **Uses:** Skin health, digestive support.

- **Preparation:** Brew tea or use as a poultice.

- **Benefits:** Astringent; may aid in wound healing.

- **Safety:** Avoid in pregnancy; internal use may cause digestive upset.

403. Yerba Mate

- **Uses:** Energy, mental clarity.

- **Preparation:** Brew as a tea.

- **Benefits:** Natural source of caffeine; may enhance focus.

- **Safety:** Limit intake; excessive use may cause digestive upset.

404. Ephedra (Ma Huang)

- **Uses:** Respiratory health, energy.

- **Preparation:** Brew tea (restricted in some regions).

- **Benefits:** Known for stimulant effects and respiratory support.

- **Safety:** Consult with caution; avoid in high doses.

405. Star Anise

- **Uses:** Digestive health, immune support.

- **Preparation:** Brew tea or use in cooking.

- **Benefits:** May aid in digestion and support immunity.

- **Safety:** Avoid Japanese star anise due to toxicity.

406. Ash Bark

- **Uses:** Joint health, digestive health.

- **Preparation:** Brew tea.

- **Benefits:** Traditionally used for joint health and digestion.

- **Safety:** Avoid in pregnancy; may cause mild digestive upset.

407. Shatavari

- **Uses:** Hormonal balance, reproductive health.

- **Preparation:** Take as a supplement or tea.

- **Benefits:** Adaptogen; may support female reproductive health.

- **Safety:** Avoid in pregnancy unless under medical guidance.

408. Cramp Bark

- **Uses:** Menstrual pain relief, muscle relaxation.

- **Preparation:** Brew tea or use tincture.

- **Benefits:** Known to relieve muscle spasms and cramps.

- **Safety:** Generally safe; consult if pregnant.

409. Blessed Thistle

- **Uses:** Digestive health, lactation support.

- **Preparation:** Brew tea.

- **Benefits:** Traditionally used to stimulate lactation and improve digestion.

- **Safety:** Avoid in pregnancy.

410. Birch Leaf

- **Uses:** Skin health, joint health.

- **Preparation:** Brew tea or use in a bath.

- **Benefits:** Traditionally used for skin issues and joint support.

- **Safety:** Generally safe; avoid in large doses.

411. Angelica Root

- **Uses:** Respiratory health, digestion.

- **Preparation:** Brew tea.

- **Benefits:** May ease respiratory issues and aid digestion.

- **Safety:** Avoid in pregnancy; may interact with medications.

412. Anise Hyssop

- **Uses:** Respiratory health, digestion.

- **Preparation:** Brew tea or use in cooking.

- **Benefits:** May support digestion and relieve respiratory issues.

- **Safety:** Generally safe; avoid in high doses.

413. Sheep Sorrel

- **Uses:** Skin health, detox.

- **Preparation:** Brew tea or use in poultice.

- **Benefits:** Known for detoxification and skin support.

- **Safety:** Avoid in high doses; may have mild laxative effects.

414. Red Root

- **Uses:** Lymphatic health, immune support.

- **Preparation:** Brew tea or take tincture.

- **Benefits:** Traditionally used to support the lymphatic system.

- **Safety:** Avoid in pregnancy; consult for prolonged use.

415. Parsley

- **Uses:** Digestive health, kidney support.

- **Preparation:** Brew tea or use in cooking.

- **Benefits:** Diuretic properties; may support kidney health.

- **Safety:** Avoid large amounts in pregnancy.

416. Burdock Root

- **Uses:** Liver support, skin health.

- **Preparation:** Brew tea or take as a supplement.

- **Benefits:** Detoxifies and supports liver function.

- **Safety:** Generally safe; may cause mild digestive upset.

417. Blue Cohosh

- **Uses:** Menstrual health, labor support.

- **Preparation:** Brew tea or take in tincture (with caution).

- **Benefits:** Traditionally used for menstrual health.

- **Safety:** Avoid during pregnancy unless under guidance.

418. Bloodroot

- **Uses:** Skin conditions, respiratory health.

- **Preparation:** Apply topically or take in small doses.

- **Benefits:** Antimicrobial properties; supports skin health.

- **Safety:** Use topically with caution; internal use may be toxic.

419. Wintergreen

- **Uses:** Pain relief, inflammation.

- **Preparation:** Topical use as oil or poultice.

- **Benefits:** Contains methyl salicylate, effective for pain relief.

- **Safety:** Avoid ingestion; toxic if used improperly.

420. Sassafras

- **Uses:** Blood purification, respiratory health.

- **Preparation:** Brew tea in small doses.

- **Benefits:** Traditionally used for respiratory and blood health.

- **Safety:** Avoid prolonged use; may contain safrole.

421. Usnea (Old Man's Beard)

- **Uses:** Immune support, wound healing.

- **Preparation:** Brew tea or apply as a poultice.

- **Benefits:** Natural antibiotic properties; supports immunity.

- **Safety:** Generally safe in moderate use.

422. Chinese Skullcap

- **Uses:** Anti-inflammatory, liver support.

- **Preparation:** Brew tea or take as a supplement.

- **Benefits:** Supports liver and reduces inflammation.

- **Safety:** Consult for prolonged use; avoid in pregnancy.

423. Coltsfoot

- **Uses:** Respiratory support, cough relief.

- **Preparation:** Brew tea.

- **Benefits:** Soothes cough and respiratory irritation.

- **Safety:** Avoid prolonged use due to liver toxicity potential.

424. Goldenseal

- **Uses:** Immune support, digestive health.

- **Preparation:** Brew tea or take in capsule form.

- **Benefits:** Known for antibacterial and anti-inflammatory properties.

- **Safety:** Avoid prolonged use; not recommended for pregnant women.

425. Fenugreek

- **Uses:** Blood sugar balance, lactation support.

- **Preparation:** Brew tea or use in cooking.

- **Benefits:** May help manage blood sugar and support milk production.

- **Safety:** Generally safe; avoid in large doses during pregnancy.

426. Cat's Claw

- **Uses:** Immune support, anti-inflammatory.

- **Preparation:** Brew tea or take in capsule form.

- **Benefits:** Known for anti-inflammatory and immune-boosting effects.

- **Safety:** Avoid during pregnancy; consult for prolonged use.

427. Gymnema Sylvestre

- **Uses:** Blood sugar regulation, weight management.

- **Preparation:** Take as a supplement.

- **Benefits:** May help curb sugar cravings and balance blood sugar.

- **Safety:** Generally safe; monitor blood sugar if diabetic.

428. Reishi Mushroom

- **Uses:** Immune support, stress relief.

- **Preparation:** Brew as tea or take as a supplement.

- **Benefits:** Adaptogen known for immune-boosting and calming effects.

- **Safety:** Generally safe; consult if on immune-suppressant medications.

429. Motherwort

- **Uses:** Heart health, menstrual support.

- **Preparation:** Brew tea or take in tincture.

- **Benefits:** May support heart function and ease menstrual symptoms.

- **Safety:** Avoid in pregnancy.

430. Artichoke Leaf

- **Uses:** Liver health, digestive aid.

- **Preparation:** Brew tea or take as a supplement.

- **Benefits:** Supports liver function and digestion.

- **Safety:** Avoid in gallstone issues; generally safe otherwise.

431. Bilberry

- **Uses:** Eye health, antioxidant support.

- **Preparation:** Brew tea or take as a supplement.

- **Benefits:** May improve eye health and circulation.

- **Safety:** Generally safe in moderate amounts.

432. Dong Quai

- **Uses:** Hormonal balance, menstrual health.

- **Preparation:** Brew tea or take in capsule form.

- **Benefits:** Known as a "female tonic"; supports menstrual cycle.

- **Safety:** Avoid during pregnancy and with blood-thinning medications.

433. Hawthorn Berries

- **Uses:** Cardiovascular health, blood pressure support.

- **Preparation:** Brew tea or take as a tincture.

- **Benefits:** May strengthen the heart and improve circulation.

- **Safety:** Consult if taking heart medications.

434. Lobelia

- **Uses:** Respiratory health, muscle relaxation.

- **Preparation:** Brew tea or use in small tincture doses.

- **Benefits:** May help clear respiratory tract and relax muscles.

- **Safety:** Toxic in high doses; use only under guidance.

435. Olive Leaf

- **Uses:** Immune support, cardiovascular health.
- **Preparation:** Brew tea or take in capsule form.
- **Benefits:** Known for antiviral and heart-supportive properties.
- **Safety:** Generally safe; consult for prolonged use.

436. Corn Silk

- **Uses:** Urinary health, bladder support.
- **Preparation:** Brew tea.
- **Benefits:** May help relieve urinary tract discomfort.
- **Safety:** Generally safe; consult if pregnant.

437. Sarsaparilla

- **Uses:** Skin health, detoxification.
- **Preparation:** Brew tea or take in capsule form.
- **Benefits:** Traditionally used for skin and as a blood purifier.
- **Safety:** Generally safe; consult for prolonged use.

438. Guggul

- **Uses:** Cholesterol management, joint support.
- **Preparation:** Take as a supplement.
- **Benefits:** Known for anti-inflammatory effects and cholesterol support.
- **Safety:** Consult if pregnant or on medication.

439. Yerba Santa

- **Uses:** Respiratory health, cough relief.
- **Preparation:** Brew tea or use in steam inhalation.

- **Benefits:** Known for clearing congestion and supporting respiratory health.

- **Safety:** Generally safe; avoid if allergic.

440. Galangal

- **Uses:** Digestive health, anti-inflammatory.

- **Preparation:** Brew tea or use in cooking.

- **Benefits:** Known for easing digestive issues and joint health.

- **Safety:** Generally safe; use with caution if sensitive to ginger.

441. Graviola (Soursop)

- **Uses:** Immune support, antioxidant.

- **Preparation:** Brew tea or take as a supplement.

- **Benefits:** Known for immune-boosting and potential anticancer properties.

- **Safety:** Consult for prolonged use; avoid during pregnancy.

442. Nettle Leaf

- **Uses:** Joint health, allergy relief.

- **Preparation:** Brew tea or use in cooking.

- **Benefits:** May help with seasonal allergies and inflammation.

- **Safety:** Generally safe; handle fresh leaves with care to avoid stinging.

443. Horehound

- **Uses:** Respiratory health, cough relief.

- **Preparation:** Brew tea or take as a syrup.

- **Benefits:** May relieve cough and support respiratory health.

- **Safety:** Avoid in pregnancy; not recommended for long-term use.

444. Greater Celandine

- **Uses:** Liver support, digestive aid.

- **Preparation:** Brew tea.

- **Benefits:** Traditionally used for liver and gallbladder health.

- **Safety:** Use cautiously; avoid in large doses or with liver conditions.

445. Hops

- **Uses:** Sleep aid, relaxation.

- **Preparation:** Brew tea or use in tincture.

- **Benefits:** May improve sleep quality and reduce anxiety.

- **Safety:** Generally safe; may cause drowsiness.

446. Kava Root

- **Uses:** Anxiety relief, relaxation.

- **Preparation:** Brew tea or take in capsule form.

- **Benefits:** Known for calming effects; often used for mild anxiety.

- **Safety:** Avoid long-term use due to liver toxicity risk.

447. Borage

- **Uses:** Skin health, adrenal support.

- **Preparation:** Brew tea or use oil topically.

- **Benefits:** Supports skin and may assist adrenal function.

- **Safety:** Avoid in pregnancy; use oil in moderation.

448. Holy Basil (Tulsi)

- **Uses:** Stress relief, immune support.

- **Preparation:** Brew tea or take as a supplement.

- **Benefits:** Adaptogen known for stress reduction and immune support.

- **Safety:** Generally safe; consult if on blood-thinning medications.

449. Gentian Root

- **Uses:** Digestive support, appetite stimulant.

- **Preparation:** Brew tea or take in tincture.

- **Benefits:** Known for supporting digestion and stimulating appetite.

- **Safety:** Avoid in stomach ulcers or acid reflux.

450. Chicory Root

- **Uses:** Digestive health, liver support.

- **Preparation:** Brew as tea or coffee substitute.

- **Benefits:** Supports digestion and liver function.

- **Safety:** Generally safe; avoid if allergic to ragweed.

451. Passionflower

- **Uses:** Sleep aid, anxiety relief.

- **Preparation:** Brew tea or use as a tincture.

- **Benefits:** Calming effects; may help with sleep and mild anxiety.

- **Safety:** May cause drowsiness; avoid with sedatives.

452. Plantain Leaf

- **Uses:** Skin healing, digestive health.

- **Preparation:** Brew tea or apply topically.

- **Benefits:** Known for soothing skin irritations and aiding digestion.

- **Safety:** Generally safe; avoid if allergic.

453. Mullein

- **Uses:** Respiratory health, ear infections.

- **Preparation:** Brew tea or make an ear oil.

- **Benefits:** Soothes respiratory tract and aids ear health.

- **Safety:** Generally safe; avoid if allergic.

454. Iceland Moss

- **Uses:** Respiratory support, digestive health.

- **Preparation:** Brew tea.

- **Benefits:** Traditionally used for respiratory issues and as a demulcent.

- **Safety:** Generally safe; avoid if allergic.

455. Schisandra Berry

- **Uses:** Liver support, energy boost.

- **Preparation:** Brew tea or take as a supplement.

- **Benefits:** Adaptogen that may enhance liver health and stamina.

- **Safety:** Consult if pregnant or on medications.

456. Alfalfa

- **Uses:** Nutrient support, joint health.

- **Preparation:** Brew tea or take as a supplement.

- **Benefits:** Rich in nutrients; supports overall wellness and joint health.

- **Safety:** Generally safe; avoid large doses during pregnancy.

457. Feverfew

- **Uses:** Migraine relief, anti-inflammatory.

- **Preparation:** Brew tea or take as a capsule.

- **Benefits:** Known for helping to reduce migraine frequency.

- **Safety:** Avoid in pregnancy; may interact with blood-thinning medications.

458. Sweet Flag (Calamus)

- **Uses:** Digestive health, respiratory support.

- **Preparation:** Brew tea or use in tincture.

- **Benefits:** Traditionally used for digestive support and congestion.

- **Safety:** Avoid long-term use; some species may be toxic.

459. Horehound

- **Uses:** Digestive health, respiratory support.

- **Preparation:** Brew tea or make syrup.

- **Benefits:** Known for easing cough and

460. Black Walnut Hull

- **Uses:** Parasitic infections, skin health.

- **Preparation:** Take as a tincture or capsule.

- **Benefits:** Known for antifungal and antiparasitic properties.

- **Safety:** Use cautiously; may cause gastrointestinal upset.

461. Dandelion Root

- **Uses:** Liver health, detoxification.

- **Preparation:** Brew tea or take as a supplement.

- **Benefits:** Supports liver function and digestion.

- **Safety:** Generally safe; may cause allergic reactions in some.

462. Mulberry

- **Uses:** Blood sugar regulation, respiratory health.

- **Preparation:** Eat fresh or brew tea from leaves.

- **Benefits:** May help lower blood sugar levels and improve respiratory health.

- **Safety:** Generally safe; avoid excessive consumption.

463. Chaste Tree (Vitex)

- **Uses:** Hormonal balance, menstrual health.

- **Preparation:** Take as a tincture or supplement.

- **Benefits:** Often used to alleviate PMS and regulate cycles.

- **Safety:** Avoid in pregnancy; consult if on hormone medications.

464. Sweet Orange Peel

- **Uses:** Digestive aid, anxiety relief.

- **Preparation:** Brew tea or use in cooking.

- **Benefits:** Known for soothing digestive issues and promoting relaxation.

- **Safety:** Generally safe; avoid excessive consumption.

465. Yerba Mate

- **Uses:** Energy boost, mental clarity.

- **Preparation:** Brew as tea.

- **Benefits:** Contains caffeine; enhances alertness and energy.

- **Safety:** Use with caution if sensitive to caffeine.

466. Ginkgo Biloba

- **Uses:** Cognitive support, circulation.

- **Preparation:** Take as a supplement or brew tea.

- **Benefits:** May improve memory and blood flow.

- **Safety:** Consult if on blood thinners; may interact with medications.

467. Gotu Kola

- **Uses:** Cognitive support, wound healing.

- **Preparation:** Brew tea or take as a supplement.

- **Benefits:** Traditionally used for mental clarity and skin healing.

- **Safety:** Generally safe; avoid excessive use.

468. Coconut Oil

- **Uses:** Skin health, digestive aid.

- **Preparation:** Use topically or consume.

- **Benefits:** Antimicrobial properties and promotes skin moisture.

- **Safety:** Generally safe; consult if allergic to coconuts.

469. Rose Hip

- **Uses:** Skin health, immune support.

- **Preparation:** Brew tea or use as oil.

- **Benefits:** High in vitamin C and antioxidants; supports skin and immunity.

- **Safety:** Generally safe; may cause digestive upset in some.

470. Thyme

- **Uses:** Respiratory health, digestive aid.

- **Preparation:** Use in cooking or brew tea.

- **Benefits:** Known for antimicrobial properties and soothing cough.

- **Safety:** Generally safe; avoid excessive amounts.

471. Astragalus Root

- **Uses:** Immune support, energy booster.

- **Preparation:** Brew tea or take as a supplement.

- **Benefits:** May enhance immune function and energy levels.

- **Safety:** Generally safe; consult if on immunosuppressants.

472. St. John's Wort

- **Uses:** Mood support, mild depression.

- **Preparation:** Brew tea or take as a supplement.

- **Benefits:** Traditionally used for enhancing mood and relieving anxiety.

- **Safety:** May interact with medications; consult before use.

473. Lavender

- **Uses:** Anxiety relief, sleep aid.

- **Preparation:** Brew tea, use essential oil, or add to bath.

- **Benefits:** Calming effects; promotes relaxation and sleep.

- **Safety:** Generally safe; use essential oils with caution.

474. Fennel Seeds

- **Uses:** Digestive health, bloating relief.

- **Preparation:** Brew tea or chew seeds.

- **Benefits:** May ease bloating and improve digestion.

- **Safety:** Generally safe; consult if pregnant.

475. Red Clover

- **Uses:** Hormonal balance, skin health.

- **Preparation:** Brew tea or take as a supplement.

- **Benefits:** Traditionally used for menopausal symptoms and skin conditions.

- **Safety:** Consult if on hormone therapy or anticoagulants.

476. Anise Seed

- **Uses:** Digestive aid, cough relief.

- **Preparation:** Brew tea or use in cooking.

- **Benefits:** Known for easing digestive discomfort and cough.

- **Safety:** Generally safe; avoid excessive amounts.

477. Cilantro

- **Uses:** Detoxification, digestive support.

- **Preparation:** Use fresh in salads or as a garnish.

- **Benefits:** May help detox heavy metals and aid digestion.

- **Safety:** Generally safe; avoid if allergic.

478. Milk Thistle

- **Uses:** Liver health, detoxification.

- **Preparation:** Take as a supplement or brew tea.

- **Benefits:** Known for supporting liver function and detoxification.

- **Safety:** Generally safe; consult if allergic to ragweed.

479. Barberry

- **Uses:** Digestive health, liver support.

- **Preparation:** Brew tea or take as a supplement.

- **Benefits:** May aid digestion and improve liver function.

- **Safety:** Consult if pregnant or taking certain medications.

480 Sea Moss

- **Uses:** Nutrient support, thyroid health.

- **Preparation:** Consume raw or as a gel in smoothies.

- **Benefits:** Rich in iodine and minerals; supports overall health.

- **Safety:** Generally safe; consult if on thyroid medication.

481. Arjuna Bark

- **Uses:** Heart health, circulation.

- **Preparation:** Brew tea or take as a supplement.

- **Benefits:** Traditionally used for heart health and improving circulation.

- **Safety:** Consult if on heart medications.

482. Wild Cherry Bark

- **Uses:** Cough relief, respiratory health.

- **Preparation:** Brew tea or take in syrup form.

- **Benefits:** Soothes cough and supports respiratory function.

- **Safety:** Use only as directed; avoid in pregnancy.

483. Moringa

- **Uses:** Nutrient support, anti-inflammatory.

- **Preparation:** Take as a supplement or add powder to smoothies.

- **Benefits:** Packed with vitamins and minerals; supports overall health.

- **Safety:** Generally safe; consult if pregnant.

484. Turmeric

- **Uses:** Anti-inflammatory, pain relief.

- **Preparation:** Use fresh, powdered in cooking, or take as a supplement.

- **Benefits:** Known for its powerful anti-inflammatory and antioxidant properties.

- **Safety:** Generally safe; consult if on anticoagulants.

485. Pomegranate

- **Uses:** Antioxidant support, cardiovascular health.

- **Preparation:** Consume fresh or as juice.

- **Benefits:** Rich in antioxidants; may improve heart health.

- **Safety:** Generally safe; consult if on certain medications.

486. Elderflower

- **Uses:** Respiratory health, immune support.

- **Preparation:** Brew tea or use in syrups.

- **Benefits:** Traditionally used for colds and flu symptoms.

- **Safety:** Generally safe; avoid excessive amounts.

487. Arugula

- **Uses:** Digestive health, nutrient support.

- **Preparation:** Use fresh in salads or cooking.

- **Benefits:** Rich in vitamins and aids digestion.

- **Safety:** Generally safe; avoid if allergic.

488. Oregano

- **Uses:** Antimicrobial, respiratory support.

- **Preparation:** Use fresh or as an oil in cooking.

- **Benefits:** Known for its antimicrobial properties and respiratory support.

- **Safety:** Generally safe; consult if allergic.

489. Black Seed Oil (Nigella Sativa)

- **Uses:** Immune support, anti-inflammatory.

- **Preparation:** Take as a supplement or oil.

- **Benefits:** Known for its immune-boosting and anti-inflammatory effects.

- **Safety:** Generally safe; consult if pregnant.

490. Raspberry Leaf

- **Uses:** Women's health, menstrual support.

- **Preparation:** Brew tea.

- **Benefits:** May ease menstrual discomfort and support pregnancy.

- **Safety:** Generally safe; avoid in the first trimester.

491. Catuaba Bark

- **Uses:** Libido enhancement, nervous system support.

- **Preparation:** Brew tea or take as a supplement.

- **Benefits:** Traditionally used as an aphrodisiac and for nervous system support.

- **Safety:** Generally safe; consult if on medications.

492. Saffron

- **Uses:** Mood enhancement, sleep support.

- **Preparation:** Use in cooking or as a supplement.

- **Benefits:** May improve mood and support sleep quality.

- **Safety:** Consult if pregnant or on antidepressants.

493. Clove

- **Uses:** Pain relief, digestive aid.

- **Preparation:** Use whole or ground in cooking; clove oil for dental pain.

- **Benefits:** Known for its analgesic properties and digestive support.

- **Safety:** Use in moderation; essential oil should be diluted.

494. Cardamom

- **Uses:** Digestive health, respiratory support.

- **Preparation:** Use in cooking or brew tea.

- **Benefits:** Aids digestion and may help with respiratory issues.

- **Safety:** Generally safe; avoid excessive amounts.

495. Kumquat

- **Uses:** Immune support, respiratory health.

- **Preparation:** Eat fresh or use in dishes.

- **Benefits:** High in vitamin C; supports overall health.

- **Safety:** Generally safe; avoid if allergic

496. Grape Seed Extract

- **Uses:** Antioxidant support, cardiovascular health.

- **Preparation:** Take as a supplement.

- **Benefits:** Rich in proanthocyanidins; may improve circulation and reduce blood pressure.

- **Safety:** Generally safe; consult if taking blood thinners.

497. Reishi Mushroom

- **Uses:** Immune support, stress relief.

- **Preparation:** Brew tea or take as a supplement.

- **Benefits:** Known for its adaptogenic properties; may enhance immune function and reduce stress.

- **Safety:** Generally safe; may cause digestive upset in some.

498. Ashitaba

- **Uses:** Nutrient boost, longevity support.

- **Preparation:** Take as a supplement or use the leaves in salads.

- **Benefits:** High in vitamins and antioxidants; traditionally used for overall health.

- **Safety:** Generally safe; consult if pregnant.

499. Catnip

- **Uses:** Digestive aid, sleep support.

- **Preparation:** Brew tea or use in herbal blends.

- **Benefits:** May relieve digestive issues and promote relaxation.

- **Safety:** Generally safe; consult if pregnant or breastfeeding.

500. Lemon Balm

- **Uses:** Anxiety relief, sleep support.

- **Preparation:** Brew tea or use in tinctures.

- **Benefits:** Known for its calming effects; may help reduce anxiety and improve sleep quality.

- **Safety:** Generally safe; avoid excessive consumption.

These remedies expand your toolkit for addressing various health issues naturally. Always consult a healthcare provider before beginning any new treatment, particularly if you are pregnant, nursing, or have existing health conditions. Individual responses to herbal remedies can vary, and safety should always be the priority.

Appendices and Resources

The following appendices and resources are designed to provide quick access to essential information on herbal remedies, including a reference guide to common herbs, dosage guidelines, recommended resources, a glossary of terms, and an index to help navigate the book effectively.

Appendix A: Quick-Reference Guide to Common Herbs and Their Uses

This guide provides a concise overview of commonly used herbs, their primary uses, and their forms of preparation.

Herb	Uses	Preparation
Chamomile	Calming, digestive aid, sleep support	Tea, tincture
Echinacea	Immune support, cold prevention	Tea, tincture, capsules
Ginger	Nausea relief, anti-inflammatory	Tea, fresh, tincture
Peppermint	Digestive aid, headache relief	Tea, essential oil, fresh leaves
Turmeric	Anti-inflammatory, antioxidant	Powder, capsules, tea
Lavender	Anxiety relief, sleep aid, skin health	Tea, essential oil, sachets
Rosemary	Memory support, digestive health	Tea, essential oil, fresh leaves
Calendula	Skin healing, anti-inflammatory	Salve, tea, tincture
Milk Thistle	Liver support, detoxification	Capsules, tea
Ashwagandha	Stress relief, energy booster	Powder, capsules

Appendix B: Dosage Guidelines for Different Herbal Preparations

Understanding dosage is critical for safety and effectiveness. Below are general dosage guidelines for various herbal preparations. Always consult with a healthcare professional before use.

Preparation Type	Dosage
Herbal Tea	1-2 teaspoons dried herb per cup of water, 2-3 times daily
Tincture	20-30 drops (1-2 mL) 2-3 times daily
Capsules	1-2 capsules (standardized extract) 1-3 times daily
Fresh Herb	1-2 tablespoons chopped herb, as needed
Essential Oils	1-2 drops diluted in a carrier oil for topical use
Salves/Creams	Apply a thin layer to the affected area as needed

Appendix C: Recommended Resources (Books, Websites, and Suppliers)

Here's a selection of books, websites, and suppliers for further exploration of herbal remedies:

Books

1. **"The Herbal Medicine-Maker's Handbook" by James Green** - A comprehensive guide to creating your own herbal remedies.

2. **"Herbal Antibiotics" by Stephen Harrod Buhner** - Focuses on the use of herbs to combat infections.

3. **"The Complete Medicinal Herbal" by Penelope Ody** - Offers insights into the properties and uses of a wide range of medicinal herbs.

4. **"The Green Pharmacy" by James A. Duke** - Discusses various herbs and their uses in treating common ailments.

Websites

- **American Herbalists Guild (www.americanherbalistsguild.com)** - A professional organization providing resources for herbal practitioners.

- **Herb Society of America (www.herbsociety.org)** - Offers educational resources and a directory of herb suppliers.

- **National Center for Complementary and Integrative Health (nccih.nih.gov)** - Provides evidence-based information on herbal supplements and their effectiveness.

Suppliers

- **Mountain Rose Herbs (www.mountainroseherbs.com)** - A trusted source for organic herbs, essential oils, and herbal supplies.

- **Herbivore Botanicals (www.herbivorebotanicals.com)** - Offers high-quality herbal skincare products.

- **Starwest Botanicals (www.starwest-botanicals.com)** - A supplier of bulk herbs and herbal products.

Appendix D: Glossary of Herbal Terms

Familiarity with herbal terminology enhances understanding and practice. Here are some common terms defined:

- **Adaptogen**: A natural substance that helps the body adapt to stress and promotes overall balance.

- **Decoction**: A method of extracting compounds from hard plant materials (such as roots) by boiling them in water.

- **Infusion**: A method of extracting compounds from softer plant materials (such as leaves and flowers) by steeping them in hot water.

- **Tincture**: A concentrated herbal extract made by soaking herbs in alcohol or vinegar.

- **Essential Oil**: Highly concentrated plant extracts that capture the plant's scent and therapeutic properties.

- **Phytochemicals**: Bioactive compounds found in plants that contribute to their medicinal properties.

- **Herbalism**: The study and practice of using plants for medicinal purposes.

References

1. Bauer, R. (2018). *Quality standards in herbal medicine*. Phytotherapy Research, 32(4), 597-610.

2. Buhner, S. H. (2012). *Herbal antibiotics: Natural alternatives for treating drug-resistant bacteria*. Storey Publishing.

3. Duke, J. A. (2009). *The green pharmacy: The ultimate compendium of herbal medicine*. St. Martin's Press.

4. Frawley, D. (2011). *The role of herbal medicine in integrative health*. Journal of Alternative and Complementary Medicine, 17(2), 101-108.

5. Foster, S., & Duke, J. A. (1990). *A field guide to medicinal plants: Eastern and central North America*. Houghton Mifflin.

6. Green, J. (2000). *The herbal medicine-maker's handbook: A home manual*. Crossing Press.

7. Hoffmann, D. (2003). *Medical herbalism: The science and practice of herbal medicine*. Healing Arts Press.

8. McIntyre, E. (2015). *Herbal healing for women: A comprehensive guide to natural remedies for women's health issues*. McGraw-Hill.

9. Ody, P. (1993). *The complete medicinal herbal: A practical guide to the healing properties of herbs*. Dorling Kindersley.

10. Petersen, R. (2016). *The herbal apothecary: 100 medicinal herbs and how to use them*. Rockridge Press.

11. Schoenfeld, D. (2019). *The herbal medicine-maker's cookbook: 75 recipes for making herbal remedies at home*. CreateSpace Independent Publishing Platform.

12. Simpson, A. (2013). *Herbal remedies: A practical guide to using herbs for health and wellness*. HarperCollins.

13. Cohen, M. H., & Eisenberg, D. M. (2002). Potential health benefits of herbal medicine: A case study in complementary and alternative medicine. *The Journal of Alternative and Complementary Medicine, 8*(3), 301-308.

14. Dahl, J. (2014). The efficacy of herbal medicine in treating common ailments. *Journal of Herbal Medicine, 4*(3), 120-129.

15. Izzo, A. A., & Ernst, E. (2009). Ethnopharmacological approaches for the study of herbal medicines: A review. *Phytotherapy Research, 23*(1), 21-39.

16. Khan, I. A., & Tazeen, S. (2012). Safety and efficacy of herbal remedies. *Journal of Pharmacy and Pharmacognosy Research, 1*(3), 75-81.

17. Lloyd, R. (2018). The importance of dosage and safety in herbal medicine. *Journal of Herbal Medicine, 8*(2), 45-52.

18. Mason, A. (2019). Growing and harvesting medicinal herbs: A practical guide. *The Herbal Academy*. Retrieved from https://theherbalacademy.com

19. Saur, A. (2021). Integrating herbal medicine into modern healthcare. *Journal of Holistic Nursing, 39*(1), 12-20.

20. Wang, L., & Zhao, Y. (2015). Phytochemical composition of common medicinal herbs. *Molecules, 20*(3), 5808-5818.

21. American Herbalists Guild. (n.d.). Retrieved from https://www.americanherbalistsguild.com

22. Herb Society of America. (n.d.). Retrieved from https://www.herbsociety.org

23. Mount Sinai Health System. (2020). Herbal remedies: A guide. Retrieved from https://www.mountsinai.org

24. National Center for Complementary and Integrative Health. (n.d.). Herbal medicine. Retrieved from https://nccih.nih.gov

25. Mayo Clinic. (2019). Herbs and supplements. Retrieved from https://www.mayoclinic.org

26. World Health Organization. (2013). WHO traditional medicine strategy 2014-2023. Retrieved from https://www.who.int

27. Barker, J. (2020). *Essential oils for beginners: The guide to getting started with essential oils.* CreateSpace Independent Publishing Platform.

28. Hansen, S. (2015). *Herbs for health and healing: 50 most effective herbs for healing & well-being.* Independently published.

29. Kowalczyk, C. (2017). *The complete guide to herbs: A comprehensive resource for creating remedies.* HarperCollins.

30. Peterson, R. (2016). *Herbal remedies: A practical guide to using herbs for health and wellness.* HarperCollins.

www.ingramcontent.com/pod-product-compliance
Lightning Source LLC
Chambersburg PA
CBHW051557250726
48653CB00004BA/1198